KETO FOR WOMEN OVER 50

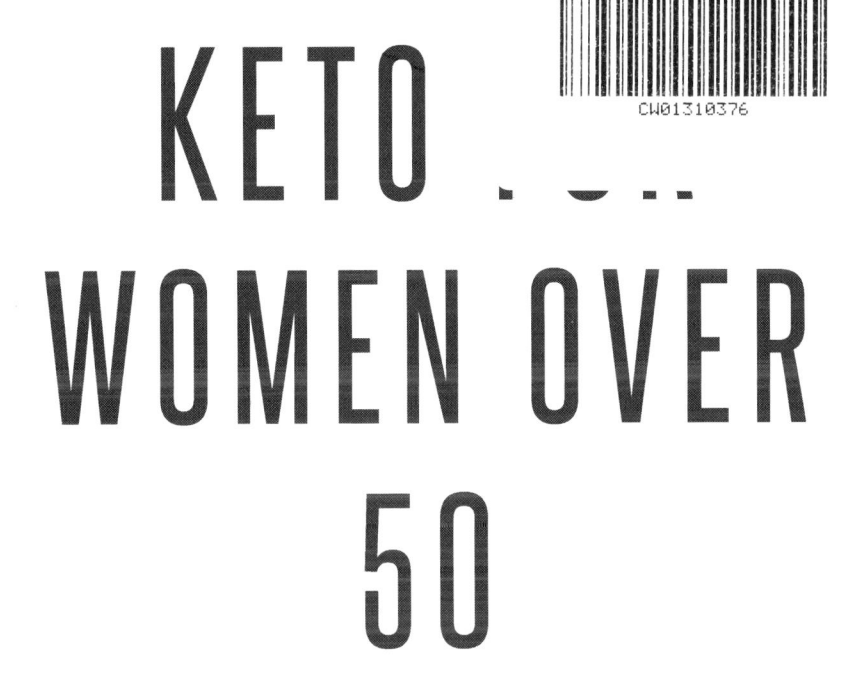

A guide to reset metabolism, burn fat, lose weight, prevent diabetes get body confidence and boost your energy with a tasty meal plan

ALICE HARWING

© **Copyright 2020 - Alice Harwing - All rights reserved.**

The content contained within this book may not be reproduced, duplicated or transmitted without direct written permission from the author or the publisher.
Under no circumstances will any blame or legal responsibility be held against the publisher, or author, for any damages, reparation, or monetary loss due to the information contained within this book. Either directly or indirectly.

Legal Notice:

This book is copyright protected. This book is only for personal use. You cannot amend, distribute, sell, use, quote or paraphrase any part, or the content within this book, without the consent of the author or publisher.

Disclaimer Notice:

Please note the information contained within this document is for educational and entertainment purposes only. All effort has been executed to present accurate, up to date, and reliable, complete information. No warranties of any kind are declared or implied. Readers acknowledge that the author is not engaging in the rendering of legal, financial, medical or professional advice. The content within this book has been derived from various sources. Please consult a licensed professional before attempting any techniques outlined in this book. By reading this document, the reader agrees that under no circumstances is the author responsible for any losses, direct or indirect, which are incurred as a result of the use of information contained within this document, including, but not limited to, — errors, omissions, or inaccuracies.

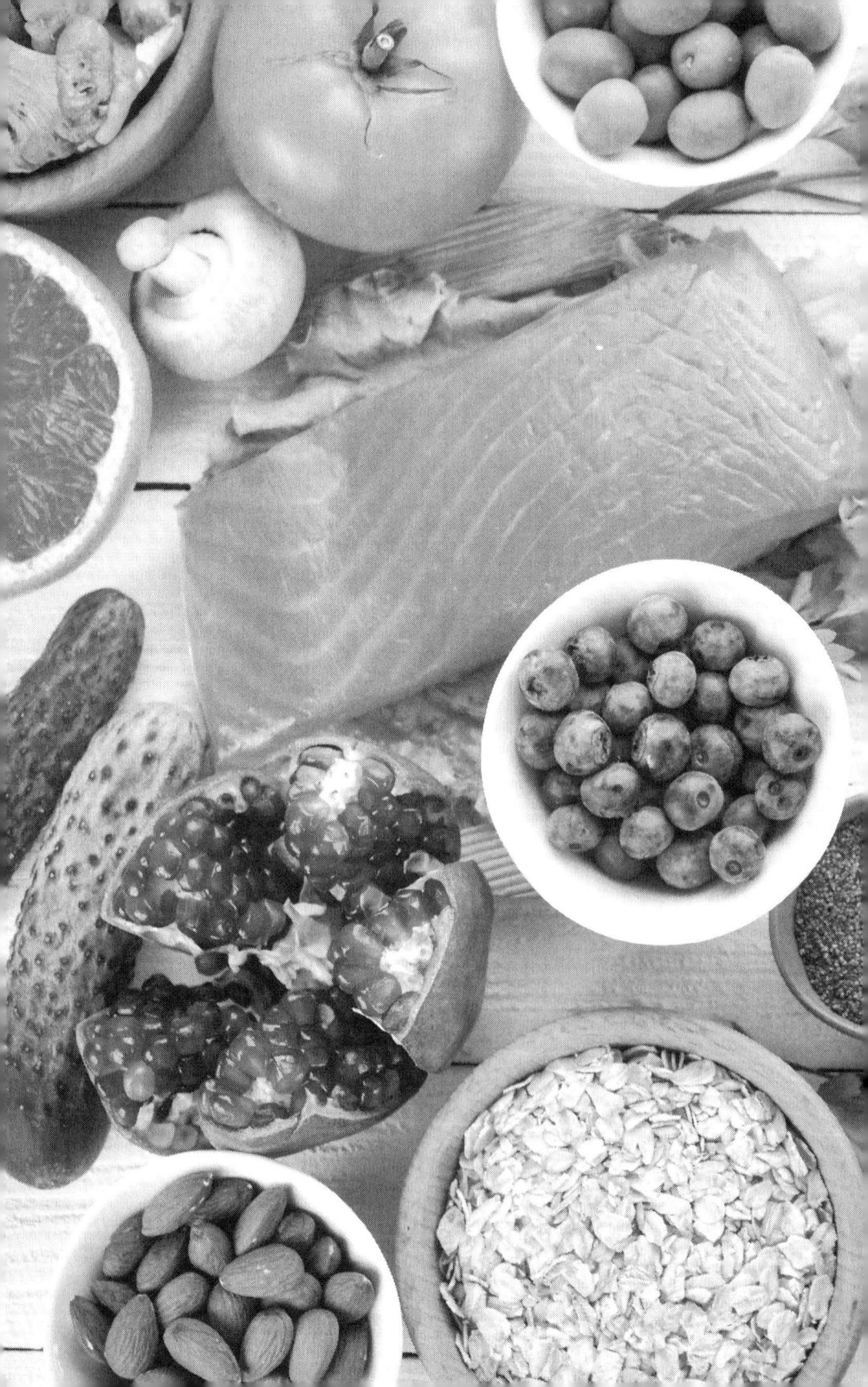

TABLE OF CONTENTS

Introduction 1

Chapter01 - What Is Ketogenic Diet and how it Works? 7

Chapter 02 - Understanding your Body 13

Chapter 03 - Changes in your Body After 50 23

Chapter 04 - Menopause 29

Chapter 05 - Benefits of Keto Diet for Women Over 50 39

Chapter 06 - Figure Out What to Eat 47

Chapter 07 - Get your Body into Ketosis and Become Fat Adapted 57

Chapter 08 - How to Have More Energy? 69

Chapter 09 - Hormone Balance 77

Chapter 10 - Keto Diet Nutrition. 30 Day Meal Plan 87

Capter 11 - How to Follow the Diet at Home and Away from Home 95

Chapter 12 - How to Keep Track of your Keto Diet 101

Chapter 13 - Tips on Losing Weight on Keto After 50 107

Chapter 14 - Conclusion 119

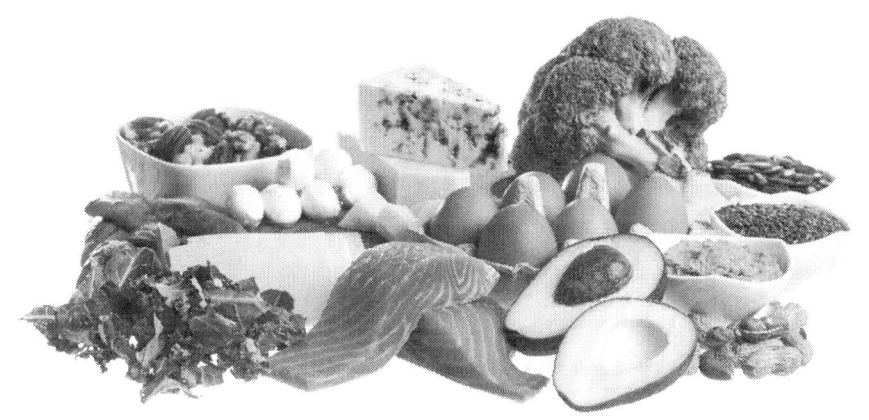

Introduction

The ketogenic diet is an "ancient" diet developed as an alternative therapy for childhood epilepsy and can now be used to promote rapid weight loss, especially in severe obesity, and to treat various pathologies, including diabetes and neurodegenerative diseases. He was born nearly 100 years ago and became popular in the 1920s and 1930s as an alternative to childhood epilepsy therapy. That is Dr. Russell Wilder of the Mayo Clinic, who theorized about the properties of this diet in 1924 and published the first scientific data on his experiments.

In the 1940s, its use in the treatment of childhood epilepsy became obsolete due to the introduction of new antiepileptics on the market. Professor Blackburn's breakthrough study from Harvard University in the 1970s began to spread and use the ketogenic diet protocol to treat obesity throughout the world.

Numerous studies have shown that the ketogenic diet can increase lose weight, improve health, and even have benefits in the treatment of diabetes, epilepsy, and Alzheimer's. There is a variety of scientific evidence about the effectiveness of the ketogenic diet in losing weight, reducing body fat and maintaining muscle mass.

Several studies have compared low-fat diets with the ketogenic diets to evaluate weight loss performance, and the results show the superiority of the ketogenic diet. A 2013 randomized study published by JCEM identified the effects of a low-carbohydrate diet on body composition and cardiovascular risk factors in 42 overweight women. It has been found that women who follow the ketogenic diet lost 2.2 times more weight than women with low calories and low fat (equal to 30%). It also shows increased levels of triglycerides and HDL (good) cholesterol.

The ketogenic diet can increase body lose weight, reduce excess fat, and increase insulin sensitivity. These are all factors that are strongly associated with type 2 diabetes, prediabetic syndrome and metabolic syndrome. Animal studies show that the ketogenic

The diet offers enormous benefits for a variety of neurodegenerative diseases, including Alzheimer's and Parkinson's disease, and can also offer protection against traumatic brain injury and stroke.

This observation is supported by studies in animal models that show how the body of ketones, especially β-hydroxybutyrate, offers nerve protection against various types of cell damage. The ketogenic diet is a dietary therapy for the treatment of epilepsy in children and, due to the reduction in insulin-related levels, can also be an excellent strategy for polycystic ovaries and acne.

INTRODUCTION

The ketogenic diet consists of a "total reorganization of the metabolism," and it is a process not without health risks: in one of the two studies; in fact, a greater propensity to obesity emerged in the mice fed a keto diet. The difference with the positive effects manifested in the other case is due to different choices made by the researchers during the experimentation phase: on the one hand, we chose to alternate the ketogenic and the regular diet, on the other the calorie intake was limited for averting weight gain.

The ketogenic diet would also improve long-term memory and longevity. For now, however, it has only been shown in mice. That ketogenic diets are now considered miraculous for weight loss is a fact, although we should always remember that for every diet we decide to follow, we should have a healthy dose of skepticism.

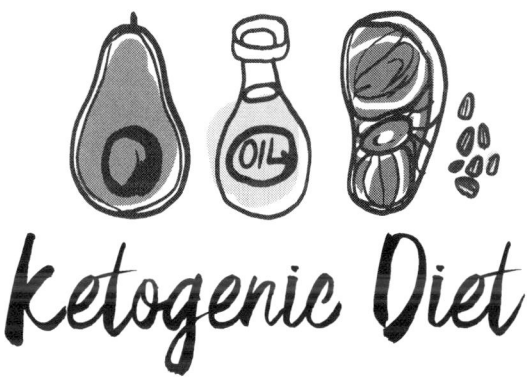

CHAPTER 01

WHAT IS KETOGENIC DIET AND HOW IT WORKS ?

Chapter 01 - What Is Ketogenic Diet and how it Works?

A diet that results in the production of ketone bodies from the liver is referred to as a ketogenic diet; it makes your system utilize fat over carbs for energy. It limits the intake of carbs to a low level causing some reactions. It's not a towering protein diet, though. It involves moderate protein, low carbs, and high-fat consumption. The precise percentage of macronutrients will vary depending on your requirements. Fat makes up 75 percent of the calories you ingest; thus is a fundamental component of the diet, proteins occupy 30% of the calories you take, and carbs make up 10%.

Your system usually works with a mixture of proteins, carbs, and fats. This diet removes carbohydrates, causing your system's stores to become depleted and the body finds an alternative source of power. Many of your organs, it can use free fatty acids, but not all of them can use ketone bodies, for instance, the brain and nervous system they can, however, use ketone bodies.

Insufficient free fatty acid disintegration releases as by-product ketone bodies. The power supplied is fat obtained non-carbohydrate, which is used by organs like the brain. As a consequence of the rapid manufacturing of ketone bodies, which makes them accumulate in the blood, ketosis develops. The manufacture and use of glucose in your system are also reduced; the protein used for power is also reduced.

The levels of glucagon and glucose are affected by ketogenic diets. Insulin transforms glucose into glycogen that is recycled as fat while glucagon transforms glycogen into glucose to provide your system with power. Carbs removal from the diet improves the levels of glucagon and decreases levels of insulin. This, in the end, causes liberation of an increased number of FFA and their decomposition in the liver that results in the manufacturing of ketone bodies and induces the ketosis state.

The diet is, in a way, identical to starvation, with the distinction being that food eaten in one. The metabolic impacts that come about and the adjustments experienced in starvation are approximately the same as those experienced during the diet. There has been an extensive study of the reaction to complete hunger, probably more so than the diet on its own. That's why the vast bulk of the information described is derived from the analyses of fasting individuals. There are few exceptions, but the diet's metabolic impacts are similar to those that occur during starvation. The reactions in ketosis as a result of carb restriction are the same as the reactions seen with starvation. In this regard, protein and fat amounts are not that important.

CHAPTER 01 - WHAT IS KETOGENIC DIET AND HOW IT WORKS?

Considering how carbs are not wanted in this diet, it may leave you wondering how much is needed for daily sustenance by your system. The body undergoes at least three significant adjustments when carbs are taken away from the diet to preserve the little glucose and protein it has. The principal adjustment is a general change in power source to FFA from glucose in most of your organs. This change spares the slight quantity of glucose accessible to power the brain. In the leukocytes, erythrocytes, and bone marrow that continue to use glucose, the second adaptation happens. These tissues break down glucose partly to lactate and pyruvate that go to the liver and are transferred back to glucose to avoid the depletion of accessible glucose reserve. Therefore, this issue doesn't end in a large decrease of glucose in your system and can be ignored in terms of the carbs need of the body. The third, and likely the most important, adjustment happens in your body, which, by the third week of continuous ketosis, transforms to the use of ketones for 75% of the power demands instead of getting from carbs. Since the brain continuously depletes glucose in the body, the regular carbohydrate demands are all that we need to bother ourselves with.

Your brain uses about 100 g of glucose daily in regular conditions. This implies that any diet that is based on fewer than 100 g of carbs daily will cause ketosis, the level of which depends on how many carbs are consumed that is the fewer carbs eaten, the greater the ketosis. Eating carbs below 100 grams will result in ketosis. With the continued adaptation of the brain to the use of ketones for a power and the glucose demands of your system decline, fewer carbs should be absorbed to sustain the ketosis state.

There is no one-size-fits-all when it comes to how much of your total calorie requirement you should derive from carbs. Some nutritionists advise that people keep it in the low end, which is five percent, but it is not necessarily good advice as the exact amount depends on your system. To get the right amount for you will have to rely on the trial and error method. Select a percentage and see how it feels for you; if you don't like the results, you can adjust accordingly. With fats and protein, just like in carbs, there is no exact amount for everyone. It all depends on you, but seventy-five percent is a good place to start off.

There is no space to' cheat' your diet here. You should follow it completely as even one meal that does not follow its rules can slow down your advancement for about a week as your body is withdrawn from ketosis. Always make sure you've eaten enough so that you will not be tempted to have a snack that could ruin all you've been working for.

Chapter 02-Understanding your Body

Metabolism

As women age, their metabolism naturally slows down by approximately 50 calories per day. This means that you need to consume fewer calories if you maintain the same level of activity.

While 50 calories may not seem like a lot, think about how long it takes and the amount of effort required to burn the same amount. According to the National Institute of Health (NIH), to lose one pound of fat per week, an average person must create a 500 calorie per day deficit. In other words, burn more calories than you consume.

As your metabolism slows down, and as we've mentioned, it could slow by 50 calories per day, it would require a deficit of 550 calories per day (or 3,850 calories per week) to lose just one pound of fat. This sounds daunting, and for many, this fact alone will cause them to give up.

MUSCLE LOSS

As people age, it is natural for both women and men to lose lean muscle mass. This has the effect of slowing the metabolism as well as lessens strength and mobility. Although there is no way to stop the body from losing muscle, the progression can be slowed with exercise, specifically resistance and strength training.

Studies have shown that when you increase your muscle mass, you boost your resting metabolism at any age. In other words, you can burn more calories while resting simply by adding weight training to your workout regimen.

If you are a woman in your fifties and have never considered building those muscles, this may be a great time to start. However, it is highly advised that you consult with your doctor before adding resistance training to your workout.

MEN VERSUS WOMEN

While it may seem that men do not experience the same weight gain/loss struggles as women, they certainly do have their struggles.

A man's metabolism slows down as well as the ages. The difference is that men do not experience the same hormonal changes, which play a major role in metabolism, weight loss, and muscle degeneration.

During menopause, when estrogen levels decrease, fat storage is promoted around. While you may have struggled your entire life with weight gain in your hips and thighs, this new fat in your belly area is not only more difficult to lose but brings with it additional health risks to your heart and organs.

Body Aches

It is natural that as you age, you are less willing to engage in physical activity. While your brain may be telling you to exercise more frequently, your body may be sending you signals that it is not ready or capable of exercise.

It is not uncommon for women to have aches and pains in their 50s and beyond that were not there just a few short years ago. From inflamed knees to achy hips and sore muscles, these body aches may hinder your ability to get out there and move. However, it is important to note that while you may have these issues NOW, they will only get worse if you do not take the initiative to exercise and manage your weight.

With added weight comes added pressure on joints and bones, making them less resilient, more inflamed, and possibly even more painful. Take control of your body and your future now to avoid many of the weight induced complications that women may experience, including diabetes, high blood pressure, certain cancers, stroke, arthritis, and heart disease.

Mental Block

For some women, weight gain has never been an issue. With an active lifestyle and healthy eating, they have always been able to maintain a healthy weight appropriate for their body type.

Unfortunately, for them, the idea that the body has shifted out of their control is a mental challenge.

Everyone has that friend. She was super skinny in high school, shapely and athletic in college, even surprisingly bounced back after giving birth to her children. Suddenly her body has decided that it no longer can maintain that metabolism level, and now that she is in her fifties, she has no way of knowing how to manage her weight.

For her, it may be a mental challenge to now have to control this part of her body that always seemed just to function properly. She never had to put any thought or effort into her eating habits or exercise routine. The fact that she now has to be concerned causes a mental block making it more difficult to maintain control of her weight.

While you may have been envious of her before, age seems to have a leveling effect. We are all going to do it! There is no avoiding it, so why not take steps to take control of your weight, manage your health, and increase your longevity.

Unfortunately, calorie counting is difficult enough, but combining this with less exercise and the natural occurrence of muscular degeneration, and you can see how women over 50 may struggle with weight loss!

The premise of this guidebook is to provide women over 50 with a healthy alternative way of eating to remain healthy and increase their chances of longevity. It also assumes that you do not suffer from health issues that may prohibit you from eating certain foods and from exercising.

CHAPTER 02-UNDERSTANDING YOUR BODY

BENEFITS OF KETO FOR WOMEN OVER 50

While the keto way of eating is beneficial for anyone at any age, for women of 50, it can have dramatic and even life-saving benefits.

Abdominal fat. Yes, I said it! There is no denying that as we age, we all tend to get a little more around the middle. Otherwise known as visceral fat, it is not only difficult to lose but increases the risk of health problems.

Keto increases fat burning, specifically targeting abdominal fat.

Insulin sensitivity. As you consume carbohydrates, they are naturally converted into glucose, which is then transported by insulin throughout the body. With age, the body's sensitivity to insulin decreases, increasing the risk of Type 2 diabetes.

Keto increases insulin sensitivity and thereby reduces the risk of developing diabetes.

Reduced inflammation. Inflammation is part of the body's natural healing process. As women age, it can occur more frequently, causing pain and discomfort.

Keto, as a high-fat diet, can have a dramatic impact on reducing inflammation.

Brain function. As the female body ages, reduced hormone levels can cause women to experience mood swings, memory loss, difficulty concentrating, and can even trigger depression and anxiety.

Keto diet provides the brain with an alternate source of fuel in ketones.

Improved cardiovascular health. Increased levels of triglycerides and "bad" cholesterol puts women over 50 at a higher risk of heart disease.

Keto is a low-carb diet that reduces triglycerides and increases "good" cholesterol, thereby reducing the risk of heart disease.

Decreased blood pressure. Although it is common for women to have lower blood pressure levels than men, it does tend to increase with age. High blood pressure brings additional risks of heart disease, stroke, and even kidney disease.

Keto is a low-carb diet, can help to reduce blood pressure.

Muscle loss. As women age, they naturally tend to lose muscle mass, which further reduces metabolism. Muscle loss can also prevent a woman from being physically active.

Keto provides a higher amount of protein, which is critical for muscle mass and to prevent loss.

Increased bone density. Women are prone to lose bone mass, which can lead to osteoporosis, the key factor in bone weakness and fracture.

Keto can help improve bone strength and density with its high levels of calcium-rich leafy greens.

Keto diet is not only beneficial to women for weight loss. However,

CHAPTER 02-UNDERSTANDING YOUR BODY

it has so many added benefits that not implementing keto as a lifestyle may be detrimental to the health of a woman over 50!

It is important to note that you should consult with your physician before starting a new diet and exercise regimen. Nothing contained in this guidebook should be considered medical advice, nor is it a guarantee that you will reap the benefits as described.

All of the recipes contained herein can be cooked in less than 30 minutes and are made with good, wholesome ingredients. Whether you are new to keto or have experience with keto, these recipes will surprise you. If you want to go keto, but do not know where to start, then this is your go-to guide. Start to lose weight and gain a healthy lifestyle today!

By considering keto to be a lifestyle, not a diet, you will be well on your way to weight loss and a living a healthier lifestyle.

KETO DIET

CHAPTER 02

CHANGES IN YOUR BODY AFTER 50

Chapter 03-Changes in your Body After 50

For women, the biggest hormonal change that happens in menopause. Menopause is a natural part that every woman experiences as a result of their aging process.

These hormone fluctuations don't only drag unpleasant symptoms with them, but they also have a serious negative effect on other hormones as well:

INSULIN

Science has found out that decreased levels of estrogen can promote insulin resistance, and in turn, increase the blood sugar. We all know that insulin is a hormone produced by the pancreas to regulate the glucose levels in our blood. When you have insulin resistance, your body is practically immune to the effects of insulin. When that happens, your cells do not open up for glucose to enter, which leaves the blood sugar endlessly traveling in the bloodstream. The pancreas then keeps producing more and more insulin to keep up with the higher glucose levels, but it is all in vain. The levels of blood sugar are elevated, and your body is resistant to insulin. This may lead to diabetes, weight gain, and many other health issues.

GHRELIN

It is known that during menopause, women experience a significant rise in the ghrelin hormone. The ghrelin hormone is also called the hunger hormone, as it stimulates the appetite and promotes the storage of body fat:

The ghrelin levels are increased. You feel hungry and trigger the reward center of the brain. Your desire for food is increased. The process of digestion speeds up and allow for calories to be absorbed much faster. The ghrelin in your gut gets released even faster.

Thanks to the rise in their ghrelin levels, women in menopause struggle with weight gain and experience an increase in abdominal fat.

These hormonal changes cause unpleasant symptoms, during, but also after the menopause transition. The decrease of estrogen may be a natural occurrence, but it puts the body through a very challenging phase of adjusting that causes mood swings, hot flashes, fatigue, insomnia, and several other fluctuations in the nervous system and brain. Some natural therapies can help women cope with these changes, but most women after 50 will tell you that maintaining weight and keeping the overall health balanced is a real struggle. The most effective way to manage the unpleasant age-related symptoms and restore the hormone balance is to rethink your diet and adopt a Ketogenic lifestyle.

Women over 50 – and those that have already been affected by menopause – besides the menopausal symptoms, in general, share three other health issues in common: low stomach acid, low thyroid function, and a sluggish gallbladder.

Low Stomach Acid

As we grow older, our stomach slows down the production of necessary acid, so most women that go through menopause do not have the adequate levels of acid for their stomachs to be functioning normally. This is an important issue that needs to be addressed. However, if thinking about starting a Ketogenic diet, low stomach acid should be specially regulated as it plays an essential role in the digestion of protein, as well as eliminating bad microbes.

Thankfully, regulating stomach acid isn't that tricky. Depending on the severity of your condition, you can restore your gut balance without any special supplements. Doctors say that simply squeezing lemon juice or sprinkling apple cider vinegar over your meat and veggies will help you pre-metabolize the food you consume, which will aid the process of digestion.

To boost the quality of your digestive juices, make sure to consume more fermented foods such as sauerkraut and kimchi, fermented drinks such as coconut kefir, and up the ginger intake.

Another trick that can help you improve stomach acid is to be mindful of consuming drinks during meals. Keep in mind that drinking plenty of water with meals only dilutes your digestive juices, so make sure to leave the hydration outside the meals.

Also, make sure to time your protein consumption. It is best to eat protein-rich foods at the beginning of the meal for better stomach acid support.

If your condition is more severe and these simple strategies don't do you much good, then you should probably take supplements half-way through mealtimes.

Low Thyroid Function

Thyroid dysfunctions are not a strange occurrence for women and are especially common for older women or those that have already started experiencing the menopause symptoms. Women over 50 often struggle with hypothyroidism (low function) and experience lower vitality, unstable mood, decrease in energy, and an increase in weight.

Choosing the Keto lifestyle itself should take care of the problem if your thyroid hormones are not significantly imbalanced. Burning fat for energy and depriving your body of glucose should make women more flexible metabolically and stabilizes their blood sugar, which should, in turn, support a balanced production of the thyroid hormones.

But if you are suffering from hypothyroidism, you shouldn't put all your money on this Keto benefit. If your thyroid hormones are not balanced, then you should also address this issue by making sure to consume an adequate amount of calories. If your body doesn't receive enough calories, it may go to a conservation state and experience a drop in the T3 thyroid hormone.

Those of you who are seriously struggling with hypothyroidism will benefit the most from a Ketogenic diet combined with carb cycling to increase the calorie intake.

CHAPTER 03-CHANGES IN YOUR BODY AFTER 50

Sluggish Gallbladder

Having a sluggish gallbladder may not seem like a particularly serious issue, but it can surely lead to many health-concerning issues. And besides, if you are willing to give the Keto diet a try, then restoring gallbladder health and bile production is a definite must. Why? Because the gallbladder is known to be the reservoir for bile, and bile being a digestive juice that helps the fat emulsion and the creation of fatty acids, you can easily connect the dots and see why it is so important when you are utilizing ketones for energy.

There are many ways in which you can improve bile production and restore your gallbladder health. Supporting the stomach acid, eating smaller meals, and staying hydrated can all do wonders for your gallbladder.

Consuming foods that are rich in chlorophyll and higher in fiber can also do the trick. Broccoli, kale sprouts, bitter herbs, and fermented foods all support gallbladder health. But perhaps the most successful natural supplement that people with sluggish gallbladder should try is MCT oil.

MCT oil is a natural product that has been refined from coconut oil. It provides a ketone source that is easy-to-digest and readily absorbed so that your liver and overall digestive tract will not have much work to do. This will relieve the stress on the gallbladder and restore its balance.

Chapter 04-Menopause

Perimenopause

Women can start experiencing hormonal changes related to menopause, years before their menopause begins. This stage is known as perimenopause, and the average age that women enter this stage is 46, but, of course, this depends on many factors and is different for every woman.

During this stage, periods become unpredictable and less frequent, and this lasts for about 5 years. This stage lasts 6 years and ends one year after the woman's last period.

Estrogen at this stage – Dips irregularly.

Menopause

Women enter menopause when they are around 51 or 52 years old. You know you are officially in menopause if one year has passed since the last period (if some other medical condition does not cause that, that is). Although the menopause symptoms, such as night sweats and hot flashes, begin in the perimenopause stage, during actual menopause, they are at its peak.

Estrogen at this stage – Drops rapidly, causing noticeable changes such as bone loss and extreme hot flashes.

Post-Menopause

Post-menopause is the stage that occurs after menopause is considered over, which varies from woman to woman. Typically, post-menopause occurs during women's 50s. And while the menopause stage is officially finished, most of the symptoms will still be there.

Estrogen at this stage – Continues to drop, which causes natural changes in the body. That may cause women to continue experiencing menopause symptoms (although not so severe) such as hot flashes.

But why does it all happen? To understand the natural changes in your body better, think of the hormones as little messengers that travel through the bloodstream and bring a dose of regulation to chemical and physical functions in our bodies. For women in their 50s, the main culprit for the change in their bodies is the ovaries.

The ovaries produce hormones that regulate the reproductive system – estrogen and progesterone. The hormones that control these two hormones are the Follicle-Stimulating Hormone (FSL) and the Luteinizing hormone (LH). At this point, we are more concerned with the FSL hormone.

CHAPTER 04 - MENOPAUSE

The FSL hormone is the messenger that sends an order of estrogen production and contributes to the release of eggs from the ovaries. When the woman reaches a certain age and enters perimenopause, her ovaries produce a decreased amount of estrogen because the ovaries have fewer eggs than during the reproductive years. But since the FSL messenger doesn't get the memo that the release order shouldn't be sent because there aren't that many eggs, this hormone gets increased. Trying to stimulate the production of estrogen, during these years, women have a higher level of the FSH hormone in their blood.

Peri-menopausal and menopausal women often describe sudden feelings of anxiety, or of being "overwhelmed," or of feeling tearful for no reason. Others report feelings of depression, and some experience rage, again, for no obvious reason.

Oestrogen is linked with the production of serotonin, one of the neurotransmitters involved in the regulation of emotions and moods.

Low serotonin is associated with low mood and confusion, high serotonin with happiness, and an increased ability to learn and carry out complex tasks. In the middle, it is calm. Very high serotonin levels result in a state similar to sedation, and very low is associated with some debilitating psychiatric conditions. Regulation of serotonin is essential for our emotional health, and most types of medication used in the treatment of depression have the effect of maintaining levels of serotonin in the blood.

Oestrogen slows down the rate at which serotonin is taken out of the bloodstream and also increases the sensitivity of the brain to serotonin by increasing the number of serotonin receptors on the brain cells.

During the "perimenopause," the levels of estrogen may rise sharply and then drop.

When estrogen rises, so do our serotonin levels. When it crashes, our serotonin levels do the same. Most of us are familiar with the effects of these types of changes as they are responsible for the emotional changes many of us experience just before a period, as estrogen levels drop dramatically (albeit temporarily).

So throughout the perimenopausal and menopausal stage, we may be experiencing the equivalent of random PMT.

Serotonin is not the only neurotransmitter involved in estrogen related mood swings. Oestrogen also slows down the rate at which both dopamine and norepinephrine are absorbed. Low estrogen results in low levels of these neurotransmitters. Dopamine is involved in regulating mood, and our feelings of reward and pleasure. Low levels lead to depressive moods.

On the other hand, very high levels of dopamine lead to feelings of aggression, irritability, impulsivity, and, ultimately, psychosis. High levels of estrogen may keep dopamine levels too high. This explains the feelings of anger and aggression that some women experience as part of PMT - estrogen levels are at their highest just before they plummet at the end of a cycle.

Norepinephrine regulates the fight and flight response to the threat, as well as alertness and energy, and at high levels produce feelings of stress and anxiety. Break it down too fast, and we are left without energy and the capacity to respond to stressful situations. If levels build-up, we may be overcome with anxiety. Oestrogen regulates the levels of norepinephrine through the same mechanism as dopamine.

As a result, during the peri-menopause, the impact of changing estrogen levels on serotonin, dopamine, and norepinephrine can result in moods that fluctuate from depression to rage.

This is, of course, the extreme. Many of us will survive with occasional feelings of anxiety or depression, and some will barely notice a difference.

What Can We Do about Mood Swings?

Exercise

Exercise is a great mood enhancer. Not only does it release endorphins, another group of neurotransmitters that give us a natural "high," but it also raises the levels of dopamine, norepinephrine, and serotonin. If your dipping estrogen levels are getting you down, exercise can help to redress the balance. Any form of exercise, a vigorous walk, or even climbing a flight of stairs, can help.

It may be the last thing you feel like doing when you are in a low mood, but it is the quickest way to correct your rebellious physiology. Most of us would not hesitate to take a pill, side effects, and all if it was going to make us feel better instantly. Exercise can do exactly that, and the side effects are all good.

If your mood has swung into an angry phase, the increased levels of serotonin brought about by exercise can calm you, and you can burn off the surplus energy of outrage.

Some people find it easier to take exercise in an organized form. You do not necessarily have to join a class. There are plenty of online courses, and YouTube is a great source of self-help videos. On the other hand, joining a class and getting involved may be exactly what you need - we are all different.

Diet

Eat a healthy diet. Go easy on caffeine, sugar, and alcohol, all of which may have effects both directly on mood, and indirectly on the important mood-regulating neurotransmitters.

Eating a healthy diet, low in processed foods, artificial colorings, salt, and sugar, can improve your energy levels and your general state of health, which will put you in a better state to deal with mood swings.

Diet is also important in helping to control or reduce your weight. How does this help with mood? Low self - esteem tends to creep in with the menopause, as a manifestation of low mood, but also as a symptom of our concerns about aging. Staving off the middle-age spread, or shedding surplus pounds can help with this. As you lose weight, exercise, with all its mood-enhancing benefits, becomes easier.

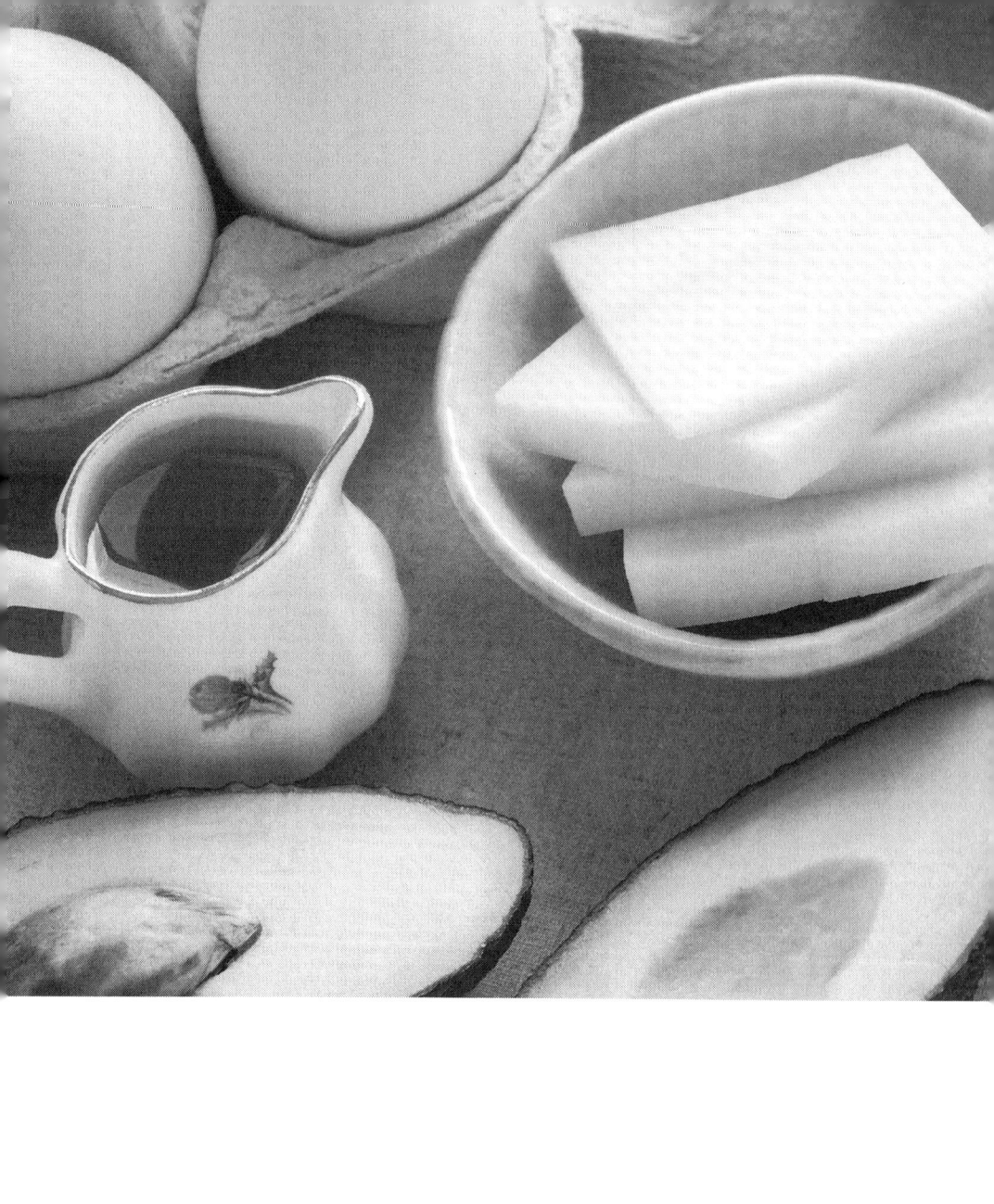

CHAPTER 05

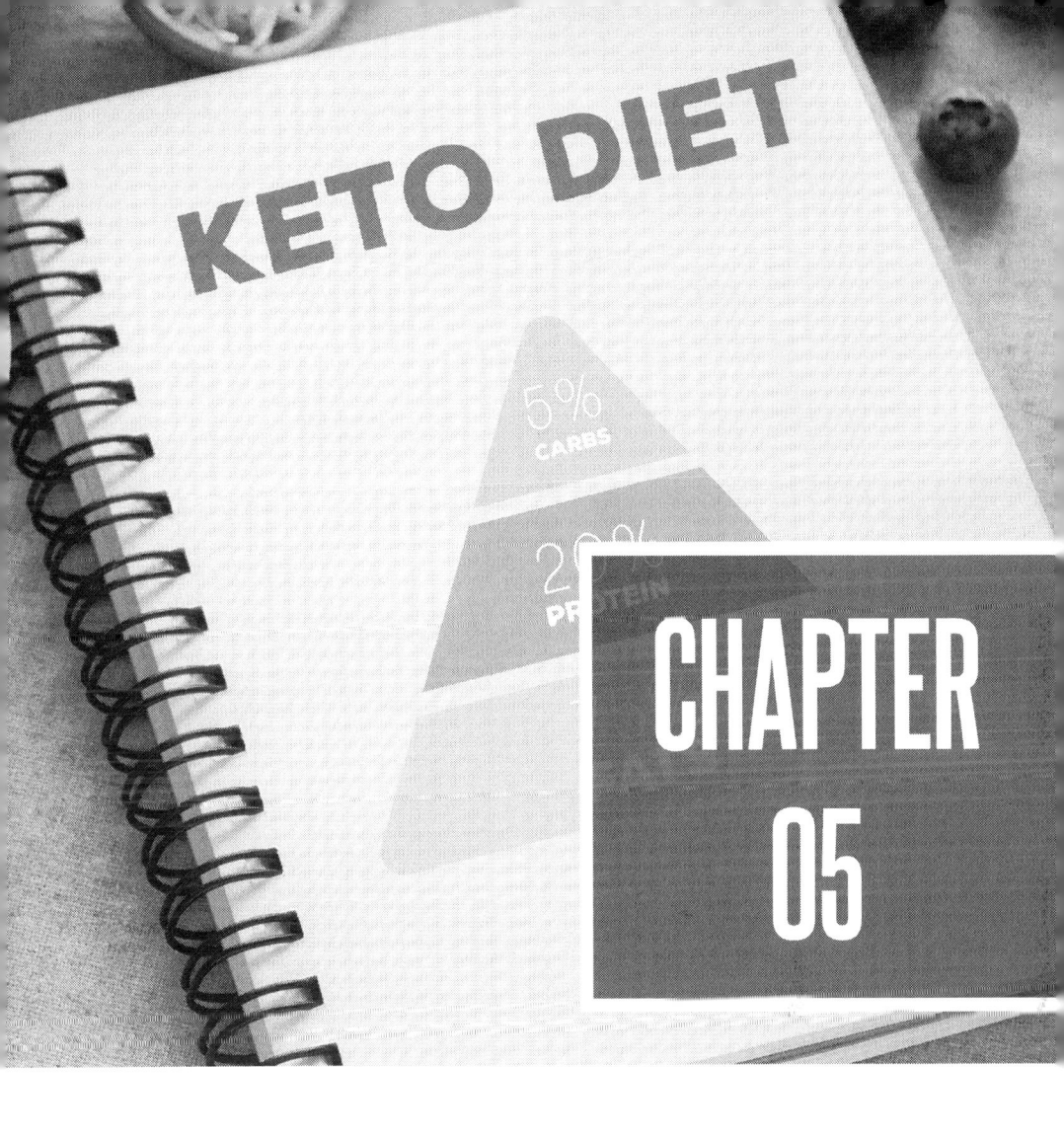

BENEFITS OF KETO DIET FOR WOMEN OVER 50

Chapter 05 - Benefits of Keto Diet for Women Over 50

Growing older is an undeniable fact of life, but it is possible to maintain a healthy and active lifestyle long into your later years. The key to doing this is to making good choices when it comes to your health, and choosing to follow the keto diet is one of the best choices you can make. Although the keto diet is good for promoting weight loss, it has so many more benefits beyond just losing a few pounds.

One benefit of the keto diet, especially in older people, is the benefits that it offers to your brain. Following the keto diet can result in a better ability to focus and an increase in overall brain function. Your brain will normally use sugar to drive its functions, but sugar has its drawbacks and is not healthy for the rest of the body. The brain can easily adapt to using ketones for fuel and function. And since the keto diet was originally invented to help control seizures in patients with epilepsy, we know it has good effects on the brain. One important side effect of the keto diet is that it seems to reduce the risk of developing Alzheimer's disease. It is believed that Alzheimer's patients suffer from increased activity in certain parts of the brain, much like people with epilepsy do, and the low carb keto diet helps to reduce the inflammation in the cells of the brain that are responsible for these conditions. And overall cognitive function and memory are enhanced in people who consume a keto diet.

Your risk of developing some form of cardiovascular disease will be greatly reduced when you begin following the keto diet. Cardiovascular disease is any disease that strikes any part of the cardiovascular system, so this includes strokes, heart attacks, high blood pressure, high cholesterol, blood clots, plaque buildup, clogged arteries, and peripheral artery disease. Cardiovascular disease can affect your entire body in some way. Carrying excess weight will cause excess fat cells to float around in your bloodstream, and this can lead to plaque buildup. Excess weight can also cause high blood pressure and high cholesterol. Losing weight will lead to a decreased risk in developing any of the forms of cardiovascular disease, and the keto diet will help you do that by making your body use stored fat for energy, which will lead to overall weight loss.

Another benefit of the keto diet in weight loss and cardiovascular health is the fact that the keto diet depends on good fats to fuel your body. The typical diet that most people consume is overloaded with saturated fats and Trans fats. You will find these types of fats in pre-packaged snack foods, processed foods, baked goods, breaded foods, and deep-fried foods. Saturated fats and Trans fats are the fats that help to hold foods together because they become solid. Think butter;

butter is a saturated fat because it is solid. The polyunsaturated fats and monounsaturated fats of the keto diet remain in their liquid state and are much healthier for your body. You will find these good fats in olives, fatty fish, avocados, and nuts and seeds, and these are all staple foods on the keto diet. Trans fats and saturated fats are the main cause of high cholesterol and high triglycerides. Since these fats are solid, think of what they probably look like inside of your arteries.

As we age, we will fall victim to inflammation. There is good inflammation that helps your body to heal when it is injured or sick. The bad inflammation comes from a poor diet and excess weight, causing excess pressure on your muscles and joints. This is what makes your joints swell and makes getting out of bed in the morning difficult. Whenever your body feels pain, it will send signals to your brain that natural pain relief is needed, and the brain sends the inflammation to the area to help heal it. When you lose weight by using the keto diet, you will eliminate much of the inflammation that you are now feeling. And the low carb aspect of the keto diet will also help to relieve inflammation because carbs cause inflammation in your body. And when you decrease the levels of inflammation in your body, you will also help to reduce or eliminate eczema, arthritis, irritable bowel syndrome, psoriasis, and acne.

The regular consumption of excess carbs will cause the elevation of particular compounds in your body that cause gout, kidney stones, and kidney disease. These compounds are usually eliminated in the urine, but if there is more than the body can eliminate, then these compounds will build up in your body. When you first start on the keto diet, the elevated ketones will cause a similar effect, but this will level out as your body flushes toxins out of your cells. After that, the levels of these compounds in your body will dramatically decrease because they will no longer have a high consumption of carbs to fuel their growth.

A diet that is high in carbs can cause gall bladder disease, which includes gall stones and blockages. When you consume food, your liver releases cholesterol, which tells the gall bladder to release bile; so that your stomach and intestines can digest your food. If you consume too much food, your liver produces too much cholesterol, and your gall bladder produces too much bile, and the result is that it will collect, unused, inside of your gall bladder and develop gall stones. When you eat a diet that is low in carbs, you will eliminate most of the cholesterol that builds up in your body. Your body makes enough cholesterol on its own and does not require more from your diet, which it gets when you consume a diet that is high in carbs. And the high-fat consumption of the keto diet will help the gall bladder to clean itself and to keep functioning properly.

The acid levels in your stomach are increased by the consumption of processed foods, sugary foods, high carb foods, grain-based foods, and certain fruits and vegetables. This increase in stomach acid leads to acid reflux, heartburn, and eventual damage to your esophagus. Your esophagus relaxes just enough to allow food to pass down into your stomach, and the muscles of the esophagus help to begin the process of digestion as they pass the food along. The band of muscles at the bottom is supposed to tighten to prevent food from coming back up. However, after years of inflammation from high carb foods, overeating, and excess stomach acid, these muscles are weakened, and stomach acid can easily travel back up your esophagus, causing heartburn and reflux. When you consume a low carb diet, you will relieve the inflammation that occurs in the esophagus and stomach and help to ease or eliminate acid reflux and heartburn.

Probably the best good side effect of the keto diet is that it will help you to lose weight since an accumulation of excess weight is responsible for almost all of the chronic illnesses that older women suffer from. Getting rid of obesity means reducing or eliminating inflammation and metabolic syndrome, which happens when your cells stop responding to the insulin that brings food to them. Metabolic syndrome is the last stage your body experiences before the onset of Type 2 Diabetes. Following the keto diet forces, your body uses its excess fat stores for energy, and this will cause the production of insulin by your pancreas to return to normal levels. And the amounts of protein and fat you will consume on the keto diet will help you to feel fuller for longer periods so that you will not be tempted to overeat or to turn to sugary treats and processed snacks.

As women age, they may experience hair loss and brittle fingernails due to a loss of collagen and biotin. The keto diet will help with both of these issues. The increased levels of protein will provide collagen and eggs, nuts, and certain low carb veggies that will provide you with biotin.

You will eat less food on the keto diet, and that may put some people off in the beginning. It might be difficult to believe that you will be able to survive on what may seem like such a small amount of food. But the carbs you have been used to eating turn to sugar in your body, and you feel the need to eat more food to keep yourself full. The keto diet relies on the consumption of healthy fats and good proteins that will fuel your body and keep you feeling full for longer than carbs will. This will lead to a reduction in the calories that you consume, which will make you lose weight and feel better. As you lose weight and decrease the amount of inflammation in your body, you will feel better and look better. And these are how the keto diet will benefit you and improve your life.

Chapter 06 - Figure Out What to Eat

Now that we have gotten to the exciting part, it is time to learn what you can and cannot eat while following your new diet. Up until this point, you have most likely followed the food pyramid stating the importance of fruits and vegetables. While they are still going to be important for vitamins and nutrients, you are going to have to be selective. Below, you will find a complete list of foods you get to enjoy on the ketogenic diet!

Keto-Friendly Vegetables

Vegetables can be tricky when you are first starting the ketogenic diet. Some vegetables hold more carbohydrates than others. The simple rule that you need to remember is above the ground is good; below the ground is bad — got that?

Some popular above-ground vegetables you should consider for your diet (starting from the least carbs to the most carbs) include:

- Spinach
- Lettuce
- Avocado
- Asparagus
- Olives
- Cucumber
- Tomato
- Eggplant
- Cabbage
- Zucchini
- Cauliflower
- Kale
- Green Beans
- Broccoli
- Peppers
- Brussel Sprouts
- And the below-ground vegetables you should avoid nclude:
- Carrots
- Onion
- Parsnip
- Beetroot
- Rutabaga
- Potato
- Sweet Potato

Every food that you put on your plate is comprised of three macronutrients: fat, protein, and carbohydrates. This will be an important lesson to learn before you begin your new diet, so be sure to take your time learning how to calculate them.

The golden rule is that meat and dairy are mostly made from protein and fat. Vegetables are mostly carbohydrates. Remember that while following the ketogenic diet, less than 5% of your calories need to come from carbohydrates. This is probably one of the trickiest tasks to get down when you are first getting started; there are hidden carbs everywhere! You will be amazed at how fast 20 grams of carbs will go in a single day, much less a single meal!

When you are first getting started, you may want to dip your toes into the carb-cutting. As a rule, vegetables that have less than 5 net carbs can be eaten fairly freely. To make them a bit more ketogenic,

I suggest putting butter on your vegetables to get a source of fat into your meal.

If you still struggle at the store, figuring out which vegetables are ketogenic, look for vegetables with leaves. Vegetables that have left are typically spinach and lettuce, both that are keto-friendly. Another rule to follow is to look for green vegetables. Generally, green vegetables like green bell peppers and green cabbage are going to be lower in carbs!

KETO-FRIENDLY FRUITS

Much like with the vegetables, many berries and fruits contain hidden carbs. As a general rule, the larger the amount of fruit, the more sugar it contains; this is why fruit is seen as nature's candy! On the ketogenic diet, that is a no go. While berries are going to be okay in moderation, it is best you leave the other fruits out for best results.

You may be thinking to yourself; I need to eat fruits for nutrients! The truth is, you can get the same nutrients from vegetables, costing you fewer carbohydrates on the ketogenic diet. While eating some berries every once in a while won't knock you out of ketosis, it is good to see how they affect you. But, if you feel like indulging in fruit as a treat, you can try some of the following:

- Raspberries
- Blackberries
- Strawberries
- Plum
- Kiwi
- Cherries
- Blueberries
- Clementine
- Cantaloupe
- Peach
- Keto-Friendly Meat

On the ketogenic diet, meat is going to become a staple for you! When you are selecting your meats, try to stick with organic, grass-fed, and unprocessed. What I do want you to keep in mind is that the ketogenic diet is not meant to be high in protein, it is meant to be high in fat. People often link the ketogenic diet to a high meat diet, and that simply is not true. As you begin your diet, there is no need to have excess amounts of meat or protein. If you do have excess protein, it is going to be converted to glucose, knocking you right out of ketosis.

There are several different proteins that you will be able to enjoy while following the ketogenic diet. When it comes to beef, you will want to try your best to stick with the fattier cuts. Some of the better cuts would include ground beef, roast, veal, and steak. If poultry is more your style, look for the darker, fattier meats. Some good options for poultry selection would be wild game, turkey, duck, quail, and good old-fashioned chicken. Other options include:

- Pork Loin
- Tenderloin
- Pork Chops
- Ham
- Bacon

On your new diet, you will also be able to enjoy several different seafood dishes! At the store, you will want to look for wild-caught sources. Some of the better options include mahi-mahi, catfish, cod, halibut, trout, sardines, salmon, tuna, and mackerel. If shellfish is more your style, you get to enjoy lobster, muscles, crab, clams, and even oysters!

Keep in mind that when selecting your meats; try to avoid the cured and processed meats. These items, such as jerky, hot dogs, salami, and pepperoni, have many artificial ingredients, additives, and unnecessary sugars that will keep you from reaching ketosis. You know the better options now, stick with them!

KETO-FRIENDLY NUTS

As you begin the ketogenic diet, there is a common misconception that you will now be able to eat as many nuts as you would like because they are high in fat. While you can enjoy a healthy serving of nuts, it is possible to go too nuts on nuts. Much like with the fruits and the vegetables, you would be surprised to learn that there are hidden carbohydrates here, too!

The lowest carb nuts you are going to find include macadamia nuts, Brazil nuts, and pecans. These are fairly low in carbohydrates and can be enjoyed freely while following the ketogenic diet. These are all great options if you are looking for a healthy, ketogenic snack or something to toss in your salad.

When you are at the shop, you will want to avoid the nuts that have been treated with glazes and sugars. All of these extra add sugar and carbohydrates, which you are going to want to avoid. The higher carb nuts include cashews, pistachios, almonds, pine, and peanuts. These nuts can be enjoyed in moderation, but it would be better to avoid.

The issue with eating nuts is that it is easy to overindulge in them. While they are technically keto-friendly, they still contain a high number of calories. With that in mind, you should only be eating when you are hungry and need energy. On the ketogenic diet, you will want to avoid snacking between meals. You don't need the nuts, but they taste good! If you want to lose weight, put the nuts down, and stick to a healthier snack instead.

Keto-Friendly Snacks

On the topic of snacks, let's take a look at keto-friendly ones to have instead of a handful of nuts! Before we begin, keep in mind that if you are looking to lose weight, you will want to avoid snacking when possible. In the beginning, it may be tougher, but as you adapt to the keto diet, your meals should keep your hunger at bay for much longer.

If you are looking for something small to take the edge off your hunger pangs, look for easy whole foods, some of these basics would include eggs, cheese, cold cuts, avocados, and even olives. As long as you have these basics in your fridge, it should stop you from reaching for the high-carb foods.

If you are looking for a snack with more of a crunch, vegetable sticks are always a great option! There are plenty of dipping sauces to add fat to your meal, as well. On top of that, pork rinds are a delicious, zero-carb treat. Beef jerky is also a good option, as long as you are aware of how many carbohydrates are in a commercial package.

With the good options in mind, it's always good to take a look at the bad. When you are snacking, avoid the high-carb fruits, the coffee with creamer, and the sugar-juices. Before you started the ketogenic diet, these were probably the easy option. You'll also want to avoid the obvious candy, chips, and donuts. Just remember when you are selecting your foods, ask if it is fueling you or not.

Keto-Friendly Oils, Sauces, and Fats

On the ketogenic diet, the key to getting enough fat into your diet is going to depend on the sauces and oils you use with your cooking. When you put enough fat into your meals, this is what is going to keep you satisfied after every meal. The secret here is to be careful with the labels. You may be surprised to learn that some of your favorite condiments may have hidden sugars (looking at you, ketchup.)

While you are going to have to be a bit more careful about your condiments, you can never go wrong with butter! Up until this point, you have probably been encouraged to consume a low-fat diet. Now, I want you to embrace the fat! You can put butter in absolutely anything! Put butter on your vegetables, stick it in your coffee, and get creative!

Oils, on the other hand, can be a bit more complicated. You see, natural oils such as fish oil, sesame oil, almond oil, ghee, pure olive oil, and even peanut oil can be used on absolutely anything. What you want to avoid are the oils that have been created in the past sixty years or so. The oils you'll want to avoid include soy oil, corn oil, sunflower oil, and any vegetable oil. Unfortunately, these oils have been highly processed and may hinder your process.

Stick with these for your diet instead:

- Butter
- Vinaigrette
- Coconut Oil
- Mayo
- Ranch Dip
- Mustard
- Guacamole
- Heavy Cream
- Thousand Island Dressing
- Salsa
- Blue Cheese Dressing
- Ranch Dip
- Pesto

When it comes to dairy, high fat is going to be your best option. Cheese and butter are great options but keep the yogurts in moderation. When it comes to milk, you will want to avoid that as there is extra sugar in milk. If you enjoy heavy cream, this can be excellent for your cooking but should be used sparingly in your coffee.

Keto-Friendly Beverages

Remember that staying hydrated, especially when you are first starting your new diet, is going to be vital! Your safest bet is to always stick with water. Whether you like your water sparkling or flat, this is always going to be a zero-carb option. If you are struggling with a headache or the keto fly, remember that you can always throw a dash of salt in there.

Chapter 07 - Get your Body into Ketosis and Become Fat Adapted

Keto-adaptation is the process in which your metabolism shifts from depending on glucose to relying mainly on fats as a source of energy. As oxidation of fats increases, your body also begins to produce ketone bodies to serve as an alternative source of fuel. Fat oxidation involves the breakdown of fats into free fatty acids. These free fatty acids are then broken down further in the liver to form ketone bodies.

The free fatty acids can be used as an energy source by almost every tissue in the body except the nervous system and brain. This is why they have to be broken down further to form ketones. The nervous system and brain need ketones to work efficiently in the absence of glucose.

This whole process of transitioning from glucose to fats and ketones does not happen overnight. Your metabolism needs some time to adjust to the new diet and energy source. You may begin to see some changes in your body within a couple of days of following the Ketogenic diet, but the adaptation process itself takes weeks.

During keto-adaptation, you will experience a delay between when you first reduce your carbohydrate consumption and having an efficient fat-burning metabolism. During this period, you will feel sick (also known as keto-flu), slow and fatigued.

Keto-flu tends to mimic the symptoms of regular flu

It is important to keep your carb intake low during keto-adaptation; otherwise, your body will not adapt as it should. Most people either give up or cheat by eating more carbs, but this will interfere with ketosis, and you will simply be prolonging the process.

There are steps you can take to minimize those initial negative effects of keto-adaptation. For now, let's look at why keto-adaptation is important and how carbohydrates interfere with the process.

The Self-Perpetuating Cycle

One of the first things you must realize is that the more carbs you consume, the more dependent you become on glucose as a source of energy. The problem with glucose is that it is utilized so fast by the body that it leaves you hungry again within a short time. As you eat more carbs to replenish your stocks, you delay your body's ability to adapt to fat-burning. But where and how does this cycle start?

Your body can store only a very small amount of glucose, and this is done in the form of glycogen. There are two types of glycogen in the body: muscle glycogen and liver glycogen. Your liver can only

CHAPTER 07 - GET YOUR BODY INTO KETOSIS AND BECOME FAT ADAPTED

store about 100 grams of glycogen while your muscles can store about 400 grams. However, the use of muscle glycogen is restricted only to the muscle that stores glycogen. For example, the glycogen in your bicep muscle can only be used by the tissues in your bicep. In other words, muscle glycogen cannot re-enter the bloodstream and travel somewhere else.

This means that liver glycogen is the only source that the body can use to stabilize your blood sugar and provide fuel for your brain. Remember that you only have 100 grams to work with, and this is a very small amount that cannot get you through the day. If your body has not yet adapted to making use of ketones for energy, you must find a way to replenish your liver glycogen. Otherwise, you will feel mentally and physically fatigued.

Estimated Energy Stores in Humans

There are two ways to get more glucose into the bloodstream. Option 1 is to eat some carbs, continue being dependent on glucose, and prevent your body from utilizing alternative sources of fuel. If you do this, you will find it very difficult to adapt to ketosis, and the negative side effects of the initial stages will be prolonged.

Option 2 is to allow your body to manufacture glucose from protein in a process known as gluconeogenesis. This process is why it is not necessary to eat carbohydrates to get glucose. The body can make its glucose in small amounts from protein, much the same way that Vitamin D is manufactured naturally by exposure to sunlight.

In other words, when you feel tired and hungry, you don't need to grab a carbohydrate meal. A lot of fats, moderate protein, and very little carbs are enough to help you make it through the day. Even after your liver glycogen runs out, there's no need to worry because your body will resort to gluconeogenesis and then ketosis to provide fuel for your needs.

One of the things you will notice during keto-adaptation is that you won't feel like eating or snacking as often as you did before. You will be able to skip meals and not feel as hungry. A Ketogenic diet can help you naturally balance your blood sugar without becoming a slave to carbohydrates.

Phases of Keto-Adaptation

Keto-adaptation generally occurs in three stages:

1. Initial Phase

During this first phase of keto-adaptation, your body will still be dependent on liver glycogen. The initial phase is very tough for most people because, to break the self-perpetuating cycle, you must stop eating carbohydrates. During this first phase, your liver glycogen stores will be dwindling, metabolism of fat will still be sub-optimal, and ketone production will be insignificant. It is safe to say that you will experience a lot of fatigue and brain fog during the first three days to two weeks.

Then there is the water loss. One aspect of the storage of glycogen is that it requires much water. Research shows that every gram of glycogen in the body requires about 3 or 4 grams of water to be stored with it. This means that as glycogen stores are depleted, you may end up losing a maximum of 2 kilograms of water! On top of that, high insulin levels usually cause water retention in the body.

Since a low-carb diet reduces insulin levels around the body, excess water can then be excreted. Therefore, you will experience drastic weight loss within the first few weeks of the Ketogenic diet.

Initially, the weight loss will primarily be excess water

However, there is one critical thing to note here. Even though you will lose water-weight during the initial phase, this will gradually decrease, and you will soon begin to lose actual fat as keto-adaptation progresses.

2. Adjustment Phase

In this second phase, your glycogen stores will have been depleted, and your body will now start making ketone bodies. Some of these ketones will be released through the urine and can be measured easily using the method described. This will enable you to confirm that you have achieved the right level of carbohydrate restriction. This phase usually takes between six and eight weeks.

During this phase, ketones are freely available as an energy source, but the levels are not yet stable enough. At this point, something quite interesting happens in the brain and muscles in regards to ketone use. When the levels of ketone bodies are still low, the muscles utilize them directly as a source of fuel, but as the levels increase, the muscles suddenly utilize them less and instead switch to fat as a fuel source. The brain, on the other hand, utilizes ketones according to their proportion in the bloodstream. When ketone levels are low, the brain only uses a small amount that allows it to function, but when ketone levels rise above a specific threshold, supply to the brain rapidly increases.

Now that there is enough supply of energy, the brain can be fully dependent on ketones, since there is no risk of running out of fuel. Your brain doesn't need you to eat frequently to work optimally, while your muscles now depend on fat to supply energy. This aspect of keto-adaptation is the one that athletes find quite valuable.

3. Maintenance phase

In this phase, your body has adapted to ketosis. The maintenance phase simply involves making the Ketogenic diet a lifestyle, and this may take up to a year or two of consistently keeping your carbs low. The aim here is to make it a habit and continue reaping the benefits for a long time to come.

Making Keto-Adaptation Easier

It is clear to see that the initial phase of keto-adaptation can be very difficult to handle for two specific reasons. The first reason is that there is very little glucose left and not enough ketone and fat metabolism to provide energy. Therefore, the best way to cope is to consume a large amount of fat. Even though your ultimate goal is to utilize body fat for energy, you must still get much fat from your diet, especially during the initial phase.

The fat will provide your body with essential nutrients and fatty

CHAPTER 07 - GET YOUR BODY INTO KETOSIS AND BECOME FAT ADAPTED

acids which are needed for producing energy. You should know by now that there is nothing to fear by eating a lot of dietary fats, so long as they're the right kind of fats.

Start by gradually increasing your intake of healthy fats

The second reason is that your body is losing a lot of water, sodium, and potassium at a very fast rate. This is responsible for fatigue, headaches, and weakness. Make sure that you consume enough sodium every day. Take about five grams or two teaspoons of table salt daily to avert these symptoms.

Table salt will help avert fatigue and headaches during keto-adaptation

You will need to get enough potassium and magnesium to prevent loss of lean muscle, cramps, dizziness, and fatigue. Meat is a good source of these minerals, but make sure that you preserve the water if you boil your meat. Potassium and magnesium tend to dissolve when meat is boiled, so use the water to make some broth.

Beef broth is a great source of mineral salts

You can also take mineral supplements to help prevent any acute effects. It is also very important that you don't forget to drink a lot of water.

Potassium and magnesium supplements will help you adapt better to ketosis

You should also ensure that you consume very little carbohydrates. If you start experimenting with your carb tolerance level at this stage, you will fail to adapt to ketosis. Make sure that you know just how much carbs your food contains. Choose a very low carb intake level (about 20 grams per day) and commit to it for as long as possible until your body starts to produce ketones. Once you know how much to eat, stick to it if you want to achieve total keto-adaptation.

CHAPTER 08

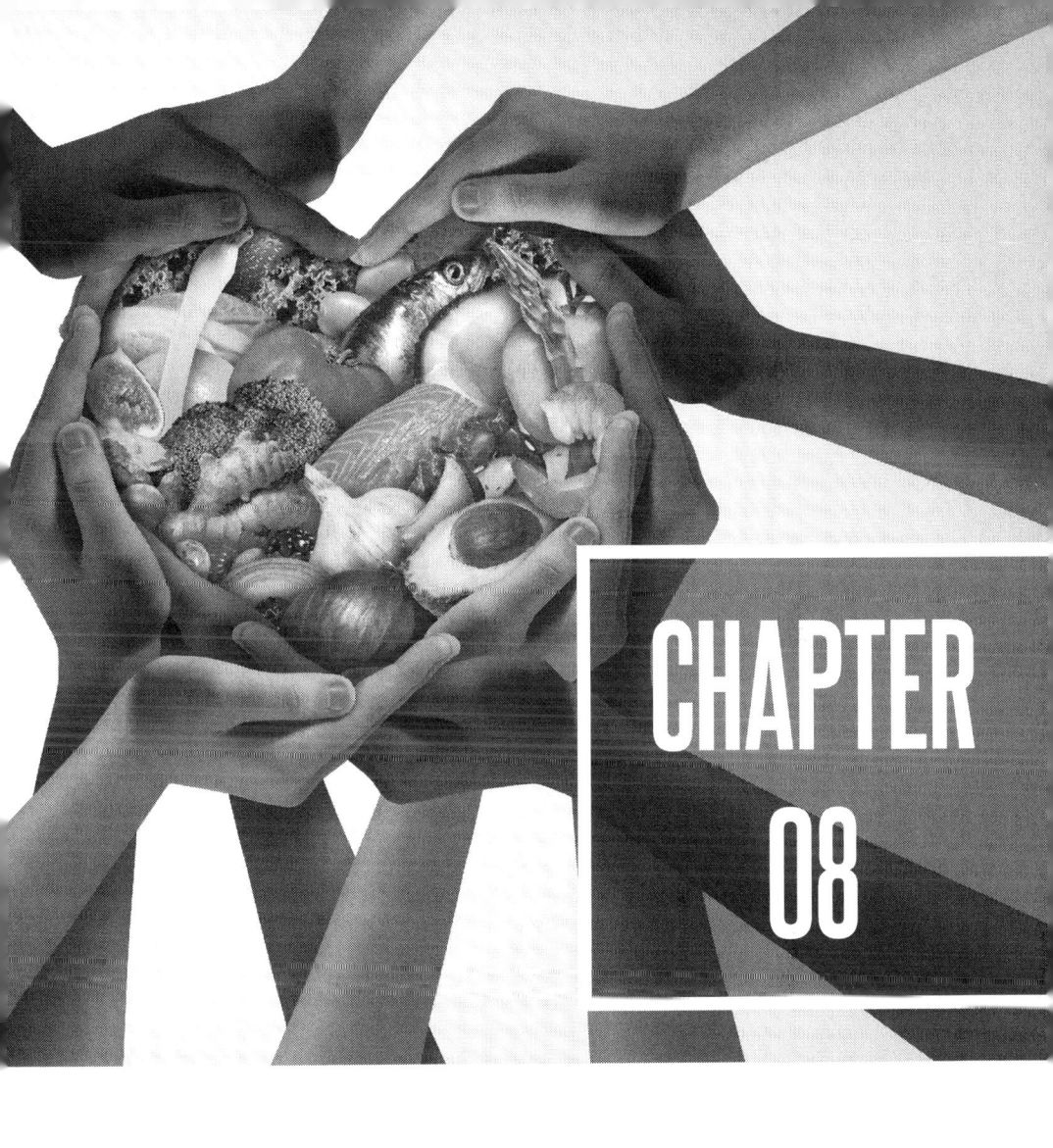

HOW TO HAVE MORE ENERGY ?

Chapter 08 - How to Have More Energy?

If feeling worn out seems to be a regular pattern in your life nowadays, this is yet another reason why trying the Keto diet can benefit you. Everyone deals with their own stressors and tasks throughout the day, but the way that the body handles all of this can differ greatly. Your food is your fuel, so it makes sense that what you put into your body is super important for making it through each day. Most of us tend to feel completely drained by the end of a long day, but this doesn't have to be your standard way of feeling. When you put the right fuel into your body, it will actually create more energy than you've ever had before.

Keto can provide you with energy that lasts, not simply bursts that are fleeting. When you only receive energy in bursts, from coffee or sugar, for example, this creates the eventual feeling of a crash. This happens because the energy is only meant to be temporary and while it can get you through a moment, it isn't going to carry you throughout your whole day. The energy that Keto can give you is the more permanent energy. It is the kind of energy that builds up gradually, preventing you from ever feeling like you are going to crash.

In the Standard American Diet (SAD), carbs are overconsumed. In general, American's eat too many simple carbs, and unhealthy fats. Most of the time, the carb takes the center of the plate, with a side of protein, and little, if any, healthy fats. Additionally, we are junk food junkies - we eat too many processed foods that are often high in carbs and sugars, eat sugared "health" foods, like sugary/syrupy yogurt, and eat out at restaurants that dish out huge servings, loaded with terrible fats, a ton of carbohydrates. Because of this high intake of the wrong kind of carbs, these starches will actually be converted into glucose or sugar molecules.

Based on your knowledge of how the body works while it is not on a Keto diet, you can gather that your body is simply going to absorb the glucose and then use that for energy. This is where the fleeting energy problem becomes very real. In order to complete this process, your body needs insulin. As your glucose levels rise, so will your insulin. Even when your body has had enough, it continues to store the extra energy (glucose) for later. The insulin will also send your body signals to your liver that the glucose stores are now full. Assuming that your body is not insulin sensitive or insulin resistant, everything should go well.

As you age, though, your body can change in a way that will make it less able to handle its insulin levels properly. When your body realizes that it needs to catch up, it will demand itself to work even harder. Sometimes, it just isn't possible for it to do so. This is when you will find that many problems arise. You might find that you have unnecessary glucose in your bloodstream. If your body isn't burning it, then it simply collects until it gets the message to do something with it. During these periods, you will likely have your biggest surges of energy. However, these are the kind that can make you very tired after only a few hours later. These spurts of energy are ultimately not useful in the long run.

It is when your body's energy levels experience these drops that you begin feeling sluggish and start to crave more sugar and carbs. Since that is what you originally gave your body for this energy that you are receiving, it is naturally going to crave more of it. If you aren't careful, this can lead to unhealthy snacking and eating habits. You might find that you are craving quick snacks to get your fix and this usually means that you are going to reach for processed or artificial foods. You do not need to have insulin resistance to experience this. It is just the way that you are training your body by the diet that you are deciding to eat.

If you feel that you can identify with these energy highs and lows, you are not alone. So many people feel this way all the time, but they do not know how to tailor their diet to truly change the pattern. For most, adjusting the carbs that are consumed is not enough. This is when you will begin to feel hungry and cranky. Eating fewer carbs without replacing them is simply telling your body that you are giving it less fuel. This will begin an internal resistance that will likely leave you feeling frustrated. At the end of the day, you will probably still want to reach for those junk food favorites.

Keto is a way for you to ensure that you are properly replacing your carbs. When you follow a Keto diet based on the given percentages, you should be getting everything that you need to keep your energy levels steady. There should be no highs and lows, only medians that you will be able to reach. By receiving energy in this way, your body isn't going to think that this is the only energy it will receive for the day. Therefore, it will not go into a state of overworking, followed by a big crash. Keto is all about balance and that is the one thing to keep in mind when you are seeking more energy.

Those who make the switch have expressed their concerns, much like concerns that you probably have. A lot of people worry that Keto just won't be enough to sustain them. They anticipate a lot of snacking and binge eating to correct this, but then they are pleasantly surprised when they realize that there is actually far less snacking needed throughout the day. When you can let go of the stigmas that surround the diet, you will find that your body will go through a natural process of adjustment. When you are changing anything, you need to make sure that you really commit to the change.

The Keto diet does drain all of your energy stores, but it replaces them with healthy fats. A lot of people assume that Keto is bad for you because it is like you are starving yourself, but that is not how it works. You are simply changing the way that your body operates and how it utilizes this energy. Your body isn't going to be angry with you for this switch like you might expect it to be. While it is an adjustment, your body is going to quickly realize that it can tap into the extra energy stores for more fuel whenever it needs to. It will learn what to do with these healthy fats that you are providing and how to make them last for long periods of time.

You will be able to say goodbye to your afternoon slumps and instead feel that you have enough energy to power through any day. There is also less of a chance that you will feel grumpy or "hangry" in-between meals. Typically, when you are between meals, your body is waiting for you to give it more energy. Since your body stores this energy when you are on a Keto diet, there are reserves for it to dip into, which truly allow you to experience your day without feeling like you are being distracted by hunger or cravings. Know that your transition into the Keto diet is going to vary. Depending on how carb-heavy your current diet is, it might take your body some time to retrain itself. For most people, it happens fairly quickly, though. You might have to deal with a few days of an unsettled stomach before you truly begin to experience the benefits of Keto, but it should not be enough to deter you.

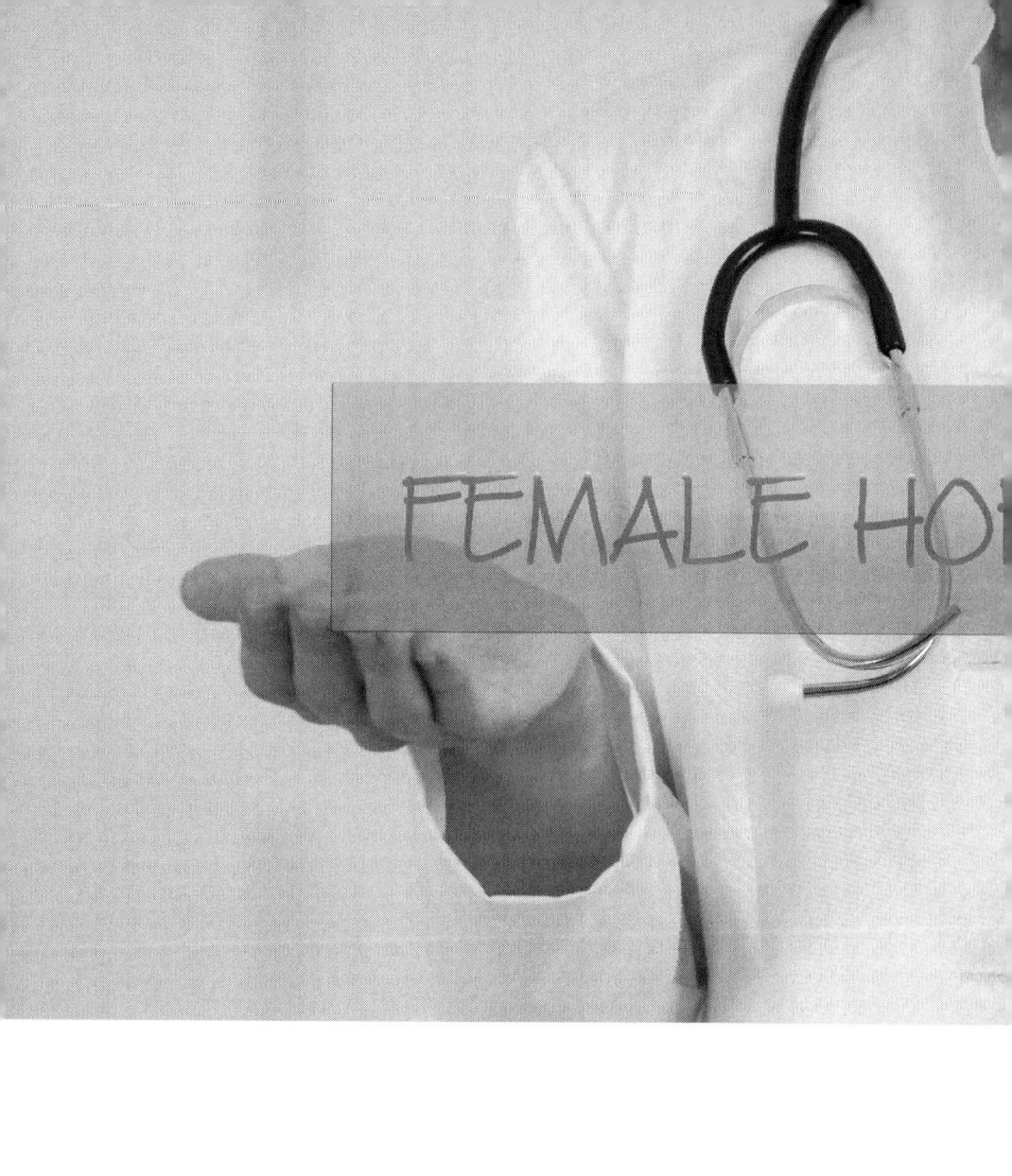

CHAPTER 09

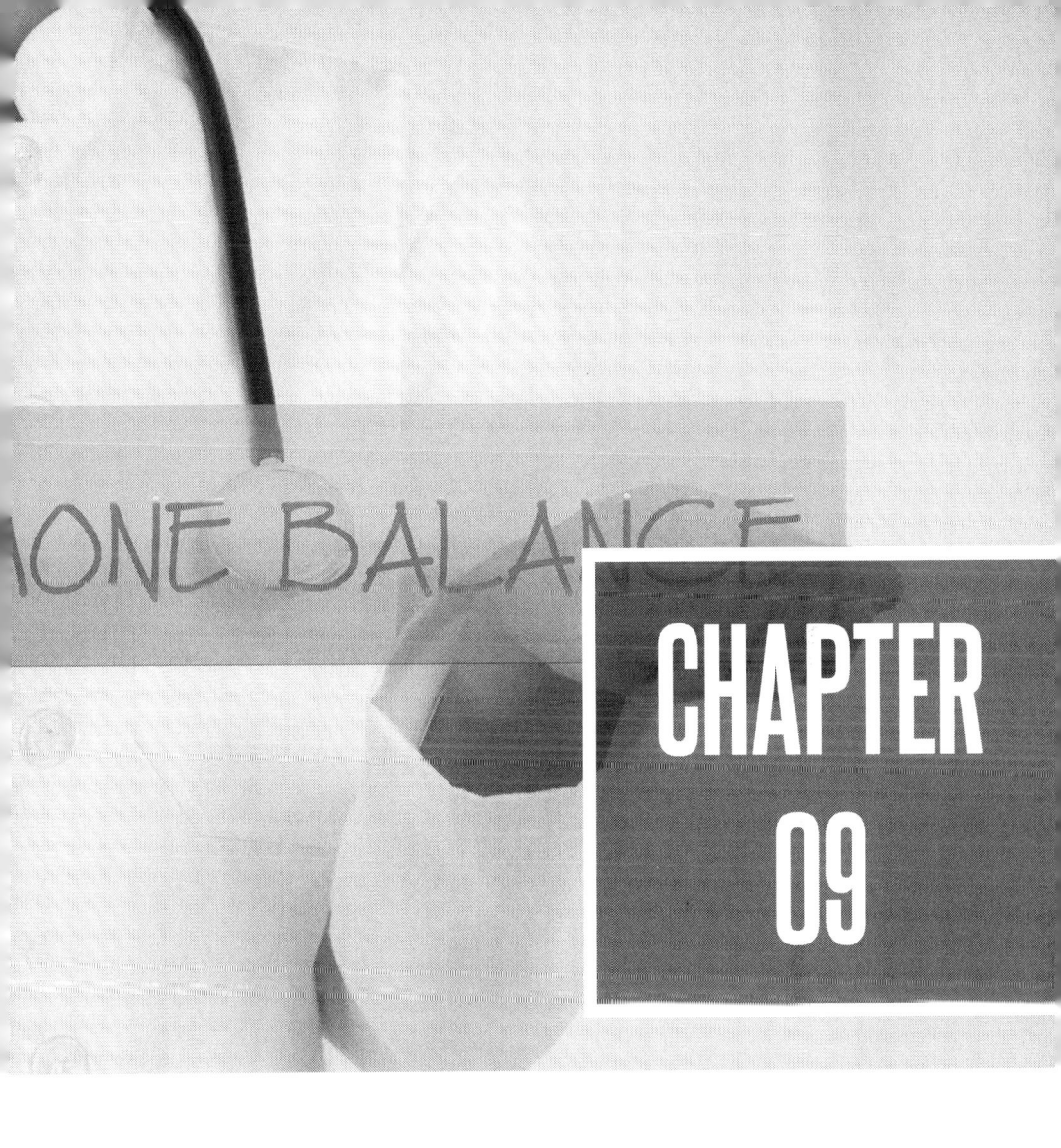

HORMONE BALANCE

Chapter 09 - Hormone Balance

With a more thorough understanding of how the ketogenic diet can help balance your hormones, it is time to learn how! By embracing the ketogenic life and applying these lessons to your everyday life, you will enjoy this diet in no time. Remember that while it will take some extra effort at first, it will be thoroughly worth it. The first thing you will want to do is focus on your diet! One of the most beneficial steps you can take is starting eating foods rich in probiotics. By doing this, you will keep your gut bacteria in check. Also, plan to eat more protein for about three days before your period, to help keep your hormones in check.

Another way you can help your hormone balance is to eat foods rich in calcium. Foods such as almonds, salmon, celery, sesame, and poppy can help with symptoms that are associated with mood swings. If you ever have questions, you can always test your hormone levels to make sure they are in check. The ones you will want to pay special attention to include cortisol, progesterone, estrogen, and SBHG. While this isn't diet-related, managing your stress levels is a vital part of balancing your hormones. Remember that stress had a major effect on your hormones, so you need to address the issue at hand. To help combat stress, remember to move your body, sleep well, and spend time with your loved ones.

Finally, you will want to test your pH levels. As we age, maintaining the alkalinity within your diet will be key. Alkalinity has a direct effect on your vitamin absorption, lowers inflammation, improved bone density, and helps you maintain a healthy weight. Luckily on the ketogenic diet, you will balance this in your diet.

Alkaline Ketogenic Diet

You are already well aware of what the ketogenic diet is, but what is an alkaline diet? We base this dieting around eating acidic foods that alter your pH balance. As you eat, your metabolism breaks down the food into metabolic waste through chemical reactions. The metabolic waste is acidic (pH under 7.0), neutral (pH of 7.0), or is alkaline (pH over 7.0). According to the alkaline diet, the pH of your metabolic waste influences your body's acidity. When your body is too acidic, this leads to health issues such as heart disease, cancer, diabetes, hypertension, and osteoporosis. To improve the acidity of your body, create an alkaline state in your body through diet.

When you create an alkaline environment in your body through the ketogenic diet, you will experience incredible benefits such as lowering inflammation within the body, balancing your hormones, and slow down the aging process. An alkaline diet can also help support your

CHAPTER 09 - HORMONE BALANCE

overall health by reducing the symptoms often in association with infertility, menopause, and PMS.

Your body is naturally alkaline. Depending on what you eat can heighten or lower your pH balance. Much like with testing ketones, you can test your pH balance through a urine testing kit. In an ideal world, you want to strive for a pH between 7.0 and 7.5. The question is, how?

The answer you are looking for is the ketogenic diet. When you combine an alkaline diet with a low-carb diet, you are lowering the number of toxic substances you are sticking in your body and providing it with more nutrients through your new diet.

To further your process, fasting is another way to keep yourself healthy and allows your body the time to take a break from the function of digesting. By doing this, your body has time to repair other parts of you and can send its energy toward helping the cells rather than digesting your dinner!

With all of this in mind, note that the ketogenic diet, while beneficial, may not completely solve your issues. Other problems can cause hormonal issues such as hypo/hyperthyroidism, over-training, stress, not eating enough, and other pre-existing hormonal balances. If you continue to struggle with your hormones, get checked out by a professional. As earlier said, there are benefits to the ketogenic diet, but it will not cure you by magic. With that being said, if it doesn't help your hormone balance, which does not mean that you will not experience others, enjoys your new diet; stick with it!

Ketosis is the ultimate goal of the ketogenic diet. It's defined as a metabolic state of greater ketone production and enhanced fat burning. But it also comes with a plethora of health bencfits. For women; however, ketosis apparently triggers a range of unpleasant side effects.

A properly executed ketogenic diet can help to restore the balance to out-of-whack female sex hormones. In my practice, I've also seen it mitigates weight gain, hot flashes, near-zero energy, low sex drive, bone loss, mood swings, and other troublesome symptoms associated with perimenopause, menopause, PMS, and post-menopause. Women who are going through major homone changes or dealing with symptoms related to homone flunctuation. I employ ketogenic nutrition to help them fix their hormones and keep them feeling healthy; especially, as they get older. Here's how and why the ketogenic diet can come to your rescue:

1. It focuses on fat for better hormone support.

Fat is your best friend on a ketogenic diet. On a true keto diet, roughly 75 percent of your calories should come from healthy fat sources; such as, avocados, nuts and seeds, coconut oil, butter, olives and olive oil, and other high-fat foods. These "good" fats support hormone production and maintain hormone balance because they are the building blocks for estrogen, progesterone, and testosterone. For too long, we've been told to be wary of fat, and thus we slashed fat in favor of carbs. This was a mistake, and personally; I believe that, this low-fat movement contributed to the hormonal challenges that many women face today.

CHAPTER 09 - HORMONE BALANCE

2. It boosts insulin sensitivity by reducing carb intake.

A keto diet restricts carbohydrates from 20 to 50 grams a day. This helps balance insulin levels. Insulin is a master hormone that controls blood sugar, and when it's too high and out of balance, your sex hormone levels can drop.

Luckily, following a ketogenic diet makes your body more "insulin sensitive." This means insulin is well-regulated, in balance, and used properly by your cells. When you're insulin sensitive, all sorts of metabolic miracles happen. You stay slim and get fit more easily; you lower your risk of cardiovascular disease, Alzheimer's disease, and dementia; you tend to not have hot flashes or night sweats; and you rebuild your bone health so that you're less at risk for frailty and osteoporosis. Cravings become a distant memory, and you feel and look healthy and energized.

3. It eases premenstrual syndrome (PMS) by detoxing the body.

PMS produces a lot of really uncomfortable symptoms, including cramps, cravings, moodiness, irritability, depression, acne, and fatigue. The underlying cause is often estrogen dominance, or having too much estrogen and not enough progesterone. One of the causes of estrogen dominance is a diet comprised of too much sugar and refined carbohydrates — a problem easily eliminated by going on a ketogenic diet.

Another cause of estrogen dominance is exposure to estrogens in the environment. These are toxic forms of estrogen that not only worsen PMS symptoms, but they are through; to increase the risk of breast cancer, endometriosis, infertility, and autoimmune diseases. In

81

my version of a keto diet, you're encouraged to eat foods that detoxify these nasty estrogens like veggies such as broccoli, cauliflower, Brussels sprouts, cabbage, and greens and delicious herbs and spices like oregano, thyme, rosemary, sage, and turmeric.

4. It boosts reproductive health by combating PCOS.

One of the main causes of infertility in women is polycystic ovary syndrome, or PCOS. This condition develops from poorly balanced sex hormones, and more than half of the women diagnosed with PCOS are obese or overweight, have poor blood sugar regulation, and have insulin resistance. There's no cure for PCOS, but because insulin problems are associated with PCOS, a ketogenic diet is a viable solution. Duke University researchers found that women with PCOS who followed a keto diet were able to balance their levels of insulin and testosterone and experience improvements in weight, infertility, and menstruation among other factors. Two women in the study got pregnant despite infertility problems, and everyone lost weight.

5. It zaps stress to protect the adrenals.

In response to life's many stressors, the adrenal glands release the hormone cortisol to galvanize energy so we can react quickly to whatever challenge we're facing. If our stress goes unresolved, the adrenals keep pumping out cortisol, resulting in too much cortisol floating around. The ongoing secretion of high amounts of cortisol robs your body of progesterone, estrogen, and testosterone, and if this keeps happening, you're more likely to experience imbalanced sex hormones, high blood sugar, loss of muscle, low sex drive, and burnout.

To combat this, enjoy all those low-carbohydrate vegetables you typically eat on a ketogenic diet (plenty of green leafy vegetables, parsley, kale, beet greens, broccoli, cauliflower, and so forth). They may help normalize cortisol, support your adrenal glands, and improve your natural progesterone levels.

The keto diet isn't for everyone, but for a lot of women in my practice it's been a game-changer for hormonal imbalance and hormone-related symptoms. If you're suffering or just not feeling your best, the keto diet is definitely worth a try!

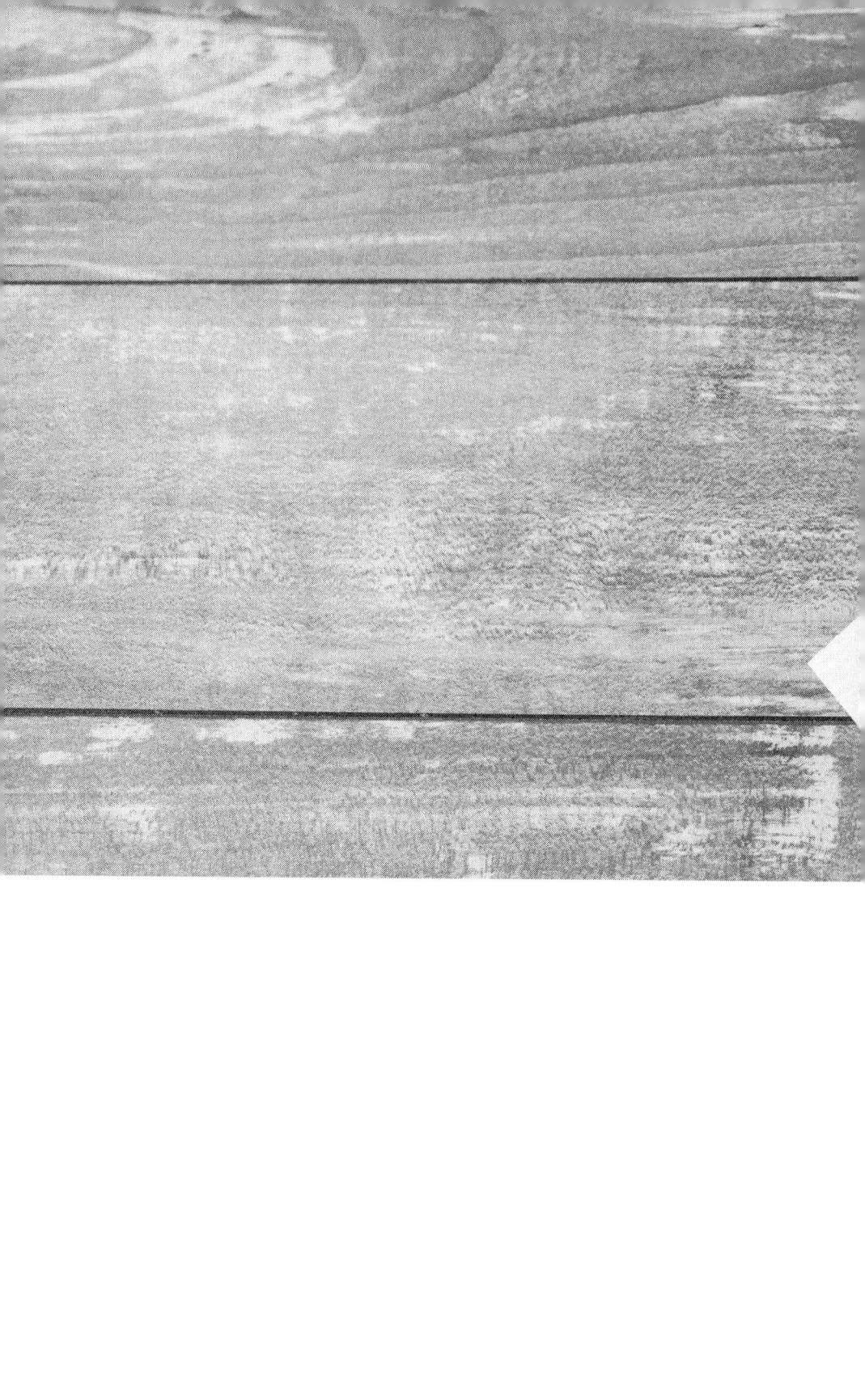

CHAPTER 10

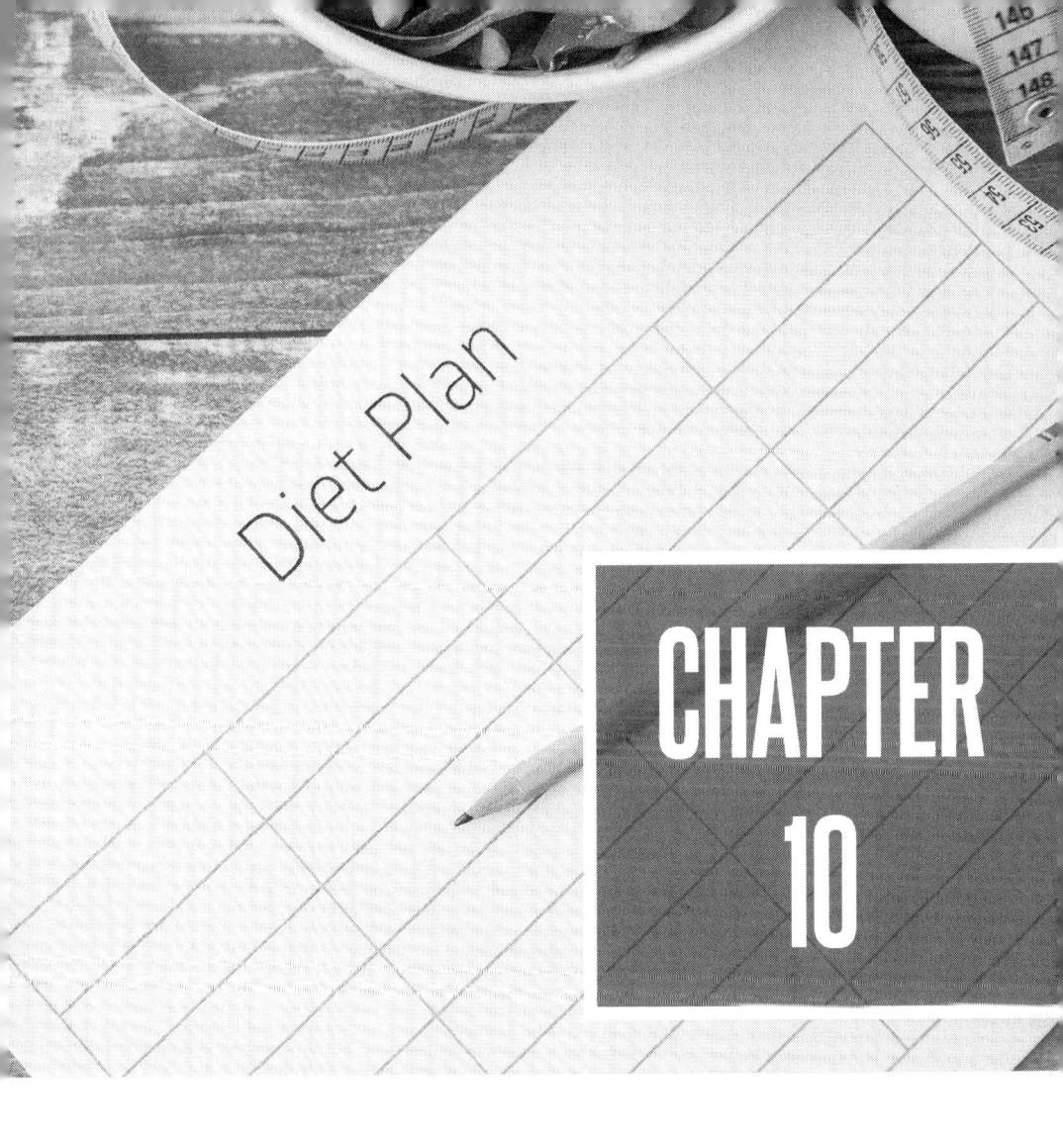

KETO DIET NUTRITION. 30 DAY MEAL PLAN

Chapter 10 - Keto Diet Nutrition. 30 Day Meal Plan

This contains a 30-day meal plan for Keto Diet to help you eat the right amount of food and keep track of daily intake. Also, to avoid the food, you should not eat in Keto diet. The meal plan will help you save a lot of time since your meal is already planned and avoids wasting food. Furthermore, the meal plan saves you a lot of money and refrain you from eating outside. The meal plan provides you a nutritionally well-balanced meal throughout the week. Meal from breakfast, lunch, dinner, and snack is provided for your convenience.

Day	Breakfast	Lunch	Dinner	Snack
1	Bacon Cheeseburger Waffles	Green Beans Salad	Korma Curry	Keto Cheesecakes
2	Keto Breakfast Cheesecake	Apple Salad	Zucchini Bars	Keto Brownies
3	Egg-Crust Pizza	Asian Salad	Mushroom Soup	Raspberry and Coconut
4	Breakfast Roll-Ups	Octopus Salad	Stuffed Portobello Mushrooms	Chocolate Pudding Delight
5	Basic Opie Rolls	Shrimp Salad	Lettuce Salad	Peanut Butter Fudge
6	Almond Coconut Egg Wraps	Lamb Salad	Onion Soup	Cinnamon Streusel Egg Loaf

CHAPTER 10 - KETO DIET NUTRITION. 30 DAY MEAL PLAN

7	Bacon & Avocado Omelet	Coconut Soup	Asparagus Salad	Snickerdoodle Muffins
8	Bacon & Cheese Frittata	Broccoli Soup	Beef with Cabbage Noodles	Yogurt and Strawberry Bowl
9	Bacon & Egg Breakfast Muffins	Simple Tomato Soup	Roast Beef and Mozzarella Plate	Sweet Cinnamon Muffin
10	Bacon Hash	Green Soup	Beef and Broccoli	Nutty Muffins
11	Bagels With Cheese	Sausage and Peppers Soup	Garlic Herb Beef Roast	Pumpkin and Cream Cheese Cup
12	Baked Apples	Avocado Soup	Sprouts Stir-fry with Kale, Broccoli, and Beef	Berries in Yogurt Cream
13	Baked Eggs In The Avocado	Avocado and Bacon Soup	Beef and Vegetable Skillet	Pumpkin Pie Mug Cake

14	Banana Pancakes	Roasted Bell Peppers Soup	Beef, Pepper and Green Beans Stir-fry	Chocolate and Strawberry Crepe
15	Breakfast Skillet	Spicy Bacon Soup	Cheesy Meatloaf	Blackberry and Coconut Flour Cupcake
16	Brunch BLT Wrap	Taco Stuffed Avocados	Roast Beef and Vegetable Plate	Keto Cheesecakes
17	Korma Curry	Buffalo Shrimp Lettuce Wraps	Breakfast Roll-Ups	Keto Brownies
18	Zucchini Bars	Keto Bacon Sushi	Basic Opie Rolls	Raspberry and Coconut
19	Mushroom Soup	Keto Burger Fat Bombs	Almond Coconut Egg Wraps	Chocolate Pudding Delight
20	Stuffed Portobello Mushrooms	Caprese Zoodles	Bacon & Avocado Omelet	Peanut Butter Fudge

CHAPTER 10 - KETO DIET NUTRITION. 30 DAY MEAL PLAN

21	Lettuce Salad	Zucchini Sushi	Bacon & Cheese Frittata	Cinnamon Streusel Egg Loaf
22	Onion Soup	Asian Chicken Lettuce Wraps	Bacon & Egg Breakfast Muffins	Snickerdoodle Muffins
23	Asparagus Salad	Prosciutto and Mozzarella Bomb	Bacon Hash	Yogurt and Strawberry Bowl
24	Beef with Cabbage Noodles	Ketofied Chick-Fil-A-style Chicken	Bagels With Cheese	Sweet Cinnamon Muffin
25	Roast Beef and Mozzarella Plate	Cheeseburger Tomatoes	Baked Apples	Nutty Muffins
26	Beef and Broccoli	Green Beans Salad	Baked Eggs In The Avocado	Pumpkin and Cream Cheese Cup
27	Garlic Herb Beef Roast	Apple Salad	Banana Pancakes	Berries in Yogurt Cream

28	Sprouts Stir-fry with Kale, Broccoli, and Beef	Asian Salad	Breakfast Skillet	Pumpkin Pie Mug Cake
29	Beef and Vegetable Skillet	Octopus Salad	Breakfast Roll-Ups	Chocolate and Strawberry Crepe
30	Beef, Pepper and Green Beans Stir-fry	Shrimp Salad	Basic Opie Rolls	Blackberry and Coconut Flour Cupcake

Capter 11 - How to Follow the Diet at Home and Away from Home

Everyone on the keto diet knows that the most available foods are not keto-friendly. There are so many foods out there that are rich in carbs but contain lots of preservatives, processed sugar and other things that harm our body. This is one of the reasons why it's so easy to get fat. Keto diet for the road might seem impossible, but it can be done. To help you, here are some tips you can stick to when on keto diet, even on the road.

Eat well before departing

Before going out, make sure you take enough of your favorite low-carb food. Don't get all too excited or in a hurry to get started on traveling. Just make sure you get enough of your fill before setting on the journey.

Keep snacks handy

This is an important aspect of keto diet, you should know. Even though keto diet keeps you energized all day and keeps you from being hungry for several hours, it is essential to keep a keto-friendly snack around when going on a journey. Nuts, hard-boiled eggs and beef jerky are some examples of snacks you can keep around for the journey. It is generally important to have a starch of keto-friendly snacks at home, at work or in your car because you never know when you might need them.

Some of my favorites include:

Mixed nuts

Hard-boiled eggs (you can get this from grocery or convenience stores).

You can also get bags of turkey/Salmon jerky/beef/chicken. However, check the sugar before buying it

You can get sting cheese, cheese pack or sliced cheese

Avocados — you can make a snack of your own by sprinkling salt on it for a satisfying and delicious snack

Canned sardine can also make a delicious keto-friendly snack

Any type of pre-cooked meat – This takes some time of planning. Rather than grilling up some burgers for your dinner, try grilling some and then wrap them in a foil to take with you

Boxed salad and dressing – This is a quick way to get some greens. You can add it with your grilled meat for a perfect lunch

CAPTER 11 - HOW TO FOLLOW THE DIET AT HOME AND AWAY FROM HOME

Peanut or almond butter and cut celery

All you have to do is to just come up with ideas for different foods and snacks that are keto-friendly. All that is important is to have something to eat on the go without any fuss. This can be essentially important when everyone eats something on the journey and you don't want to feel left out.

Pre-made lunches

The importance of pre-made lunches cannot be overemphasized. You can make it super-fancy or just simple. One of the keys to successful dieting is pre-made lunches. As with the above where you get to grill some meats, you could do the same, and buy a box of salad and dressing. You can eat them for the entire week. You can just add avocado, cucumber, hard-boiled eggs, mushrooms or salted asparagus and any seasonal vegetables. You can add something to make it feel like a gourmet, such as beef jerky. Make sure to check that your salad dressing does not contain lots of carbs or sugar (ranch, oil vinegar, blue cheese can also work).

Other nice options are:

celery and bun-less cheeseburgers and dressing

grilled Portobello mushrooms and chicken thighs

Tuna salad lettuce cups

keto friendly sandwiches — meat, bacon, cheese, avocado and mustard between red lettuce or romaine

Fast food options and Eating out

Many people often complain that their keto diet makes it difficult to eat out, but this is not so true. You can eat out by simply cutting out the carbs. For instance, ordering a burger or sandwich which comes with chips or French fries. You can substitute lettuce for buns or rather, you can ask for it to be served on a bed of greens. You can also request salad instead of taters. Although some restaurants might sell the salad to you, it's just a little price to pay to stick to your diet.

For breakfast, you can do the same. You can substitute salad for toast in addition to your omelet. Instead of hash browns, you can request sautéed or grilled vegetables. And for dinner, you can replace bread with lettuce and substitute all the starch with vegetables.

When traveling and you make the stop to get some food in a restaurant, you probably know already that many places are better at serving burgers on top of lettuce or with lettuce buns. If the restaurant doesn't take the buns out of the sandwich, you can simply take it off yourself. Make sure you avoid chicken nuggets because they certainly contain carbs and are not keto-friendly.

Cheat days

It is not advisable to cheat on your diet more than once in a week, but at least you are allowed to cheat sometimes on a trip. This is one of the best parts of keto diet; it lets you cheat now and then as far as you get back to it as quickly as possible. So in times of a night out with some friends for some pizza and beer, you can go ahead. In the morning, be prepared to get back on your diet. As far as you do it, your body will be back in ketosis soon enough.

Learn to fast

Fasting is one of the most difficult parts of keto diet, but it remains a very effective aspect. If you are just getting started on keto diet, fasting is not yet suitable for you. In the beginning, you just have to pay attention to getting enough to eat so you won't be super hungry.

As you stick to the diet, with time, you will notice you are not as hungry as you used to be. At this point, you can start fasting. An easy way to fast is to make use of the time you are sleeping as a starting point. When morning comes, get a coffee and in the middle of the day, you can treat yourself to a little snack like some nuts and hard-boiled eggs. You can fast with your snacks the next day. After that, you can wait until lunch before having a whole meal. With this, you have fasted for 42 hours, which is not bad.

Several researches showed many benefits of intermittent fasting. Even if all you can do is fast for just 15 to 20 hours, it's still enough. The best time length for fasting for health purposes is three days. It is believed that fasting for this duration several times in a year helps to prevent cancer.

The best thing about the fast is that you don't have to treat it as a serious fast more than once a month, especially the moment you get into the rotation of 15 to 20 hours fast now and then. If you are used to eating three to four times per day, you will have a lot of work on your hands. However, if you can learn to fast, then it will be a powerful tool that can help you achieve your goal.

Chapter 12 - How to Keep Track of your Keto Diet

Keeping track of your Keto diet is something that is important and will go a long way towards your success. The first thing that you have probably noticed is that the eBook has already talked a little about tracking what you are doing with measuring your ketones. This is something that is important, but there is so much more to the diet than just eliminating carbs and increasing your protein and high-fat content. This is, unfortunately, an oversimplification of the diet, but that's the bad news, the good news is when you keep track of the diet you will be able to discern the relationships between the different types of food that you are consuming and how it affects not just how you get into the state of ketosis but how you feel when you eat these foods. The goal of the diet is for you to lose weight and feel great, so if you are losing weight but you are not feeling great, then something is wrong, and it needs to be fixed so that it why tracking what you are doing is so very important. Make sure that you are detailed in your tracking of what you do so that you can be sure that you are getting the most out of your Keto Diet. Focusing on things like the percentages along with the foods you ate and what times is a great place to start.

Naturally, there are questions about how to track your progress, but the good news is the techniques that are out there for tracking your progress come down to repetition and being detailed. The more you can add, the better you will do. Now, before we get into a longer discussion about the things to track and how to track them, what you need to know is that there are a ton of apps out there that will help you keep track of your progress on the Keto Diet and help you make sure that you are not straying outside the lines with how you are working your specific ration. The good news is that these apps can go on your smartphone, and you can carry them around with you to have you in a better position for making sure that you are sticking with your diet. There are a few things that are important to track, though, and they are signposts for how well you are doing on the Keto Diet.

Weight Loss

The most important thing that you can track with the Keto Diet is your weight loss. This is the critical component of the diet and the ultimate end goal. There are several ways that you can track your weight loss, but the first thing you need to do is get a scale. The good news is you do not need a scale that does all sorts of things like measure body fat and whatnot; instead, you can get a scale that will simply display your weight. These scales are relatively cheap and are at every single major store.

Once you have your scale, the next thing to do is weigh yourself. The key to weighing yourself is to do so every single day at the same time and under the same circumstances. The best way to track your weight is to weigh yourself in the morning when you wake up, but after you have gone to the bathroom. This is when you are at your

CHAPTER 12 - HOW TO KEEP TRACK OF YOUR KETO DIET

most accurate weight because your body has gotten rid of most of its excess weight. Check your weight. There are several things to do here. You could record your weight on the app that you chose to track your progress on the Keto Diet, or you could keep a chart. One really helpful thing is the social promotion aspect of how you are losing weight. Posting your weight every day on social media will get people that are in your life to rally around you and provide encouragement. It also helps you stay on top of your game. The last thing that you want is to be in a position where you want to get out of the diet. So keeping track of your weight is especially important because it ensures that you are sticking with the diet and making sure the diet is doing exactly what you need it to do – keeping you healthy and losing weight.

As you use the programs to track your weight, track other changes as well. Take your measurements. What is your waist size and your chest size? This is where bad fat gets stored, so if you know what your size is. You do your measurements every couple weeks, and this is another way to give yourself the positive reinforcement you need to make sure that you are doing what needs to be done to lose the weight and keep it off when getting on the Keto Diet.

Tracking your Food

This is something else that is important – you have to keep track of what you eat with the Keto Diet. This matters because as you eat the food, you are also going to be testing your levels of ketones in your body. When you do a food diary, this is a great way to make sure that you are doing the right levels of calories along with the different grams of food that you need to eat. There are so many different things to do with a food diary, but when you keep a food diary, what ends up happening is that you can correlate how you are feeling and your levels of ketones with what you are eating. This, in turn, makes your time on the Keto Diet that much more productive – you can lose weight with greater efficiency, and in turn that make it so that you can easily keep yourself faithful to the diet. Having a food journal is easy to do, and it is found on many of the Keto Diet apps.

Tracking your Ketones

The other thing that people on the Keto Diet need to do is stay abreast of where their numbers are. Now when it comes to testing yourself, doing stuff like taking a blood test is something that you should not do every day because you will not see much variance. However, if you want to make sure that each day you are doing a little bit better, it is very easy to use the tools such as the breath analyzer and the urine strips. These tools make it so easy to check your levels of ketones, see if you are in ketosis, and at the end of the day, make sure that you are doing what is necessary to keep yourself in this state in conjunction with the food that you are eating and the substances you are drinking.

That being said, the initial foray into ketosis is not the easiest thing, so that requires a lot of patience. With all of the different Keto Diet apps that are out there, you can be sure to input the readings, and some of the different devices are even able to integrate with the apps, which makes them that much more formidable when it comes to keeping track of all the different things that you are doing. The bottom line is that as long as you are getting the numbers that you need to see and that they are heading in the right direction, you can rest assured that it will be quite simple to get to the point where your body is burning

CHAPTER 12 - HOW TO KEEP TRACK OF YOUR KETO DIET

your fat cells instead of looking for the different glycogen stores – because those glycogen stores are not there.

When it comes to tracking what you do, it is always better to be disciplined and vigilant with your tracking. This is the simplest way to make sure that what you are doing is producing results. The worst thing would be if you are trying to keep track of stuff, but at the same time, you are not able to correlate the data with the outcomes. The Keto Diet does require a massive amount of cohesion with all of the different elements, and that is why this is not the easiest of diets, but when you are keeping track of everything that you are doing, what ends up happening is that the diet becomes a rewarding endeavor and the signposts that you get from the tracking are things that keep you engaged with the diet and pushing yourself to greater heights for weighing that you can lose along with being that much more healthy. So, find a Keto Diet app that you like and get started right away with tracking all the different parts of the diet.

Chapter 13 - Tips on Losing Weight on Keto After 50

EXERCISE

In the fitness world, it is already established that 80% of your weight loss success comes from the diet. So just by following the keto diet alone, you are already making great progress. However, if you want that extra edge in your weight loss, consider doing exercises.

You have plenty of options here. You can do cardio exercises such as jogging, running, or cycling every morning for 30 minutes, but strength training works just as well for older adults. You should do both if you can.

Cardio exercises can get the heart pumping and get the body moving more freely, but note that your muscle mass starts to decline after 50. So work on your muscles as well.

How much exercise should you do? It depends on how much you can handle. No point in pushing beyond the limit and regret it later, right?

Team Up

A group activity is always more entertaining. So if you can find like-minded individuals who are also into keto diets, consider doing it together with them. It makes things much easier. This tip also applies to some other tips that I will show you, such as exercise that I just covered.

Move More

Moving more here does not mean more cardio exercises. You cannot expect to get any more effective weight loss if you exercise for 30mns a day and then sit on the couch for the rest of the day. The idea is to burn more calories than you can take in, so it pays to be a little extra active throughout the day.

If you have a desk job, consider getting up at least once an hour and take a short break by walking in the lobby for at least 5 minutes. It doesn't seem much, but it helps in the long run.

More Protein

Protein is very important for both weight loss and youth, including the protection against muscle degradation and other aging ailments.

Couple a high protein intake with strength exercise, and you can be sure that you would be building muscles faster than they can degrade. You won't look like Arnold when he was a bodybuilder, but you might even look fitter than the guy in his 20s at your workplace.

Talk to a Dietitian

The first thing you should do before getting into any diet is to consult your dietitian. While the keto diet works for many people, you never really know if it will work for you. Therefore, it is wise to ask your dietitian first before you jump in, rather than suffer some adverse effects because your body is not compatible with this diet.

Cook at Home More

Or eat out less frequently. There are two reasons why you should do that. For one, there are only a few places, if at all, that serve keto-based foods, let alone those that follow your diet plan. You need to prepare your food if you want to do a keto diet. Another benefit is economics. You will buy most of your ingredients and prepare your meals ahead of time. This means you will only spend your money on the ingredients you know you will need.

Eat More Produce

While we are on the subject of eating, consider incorporating more produces in your diet, some of which I have covered already. Vegetables and fruits are full of nutrients that your body needs to remain healthy, so it should be included in your diet.

A Personal Trainer

While we are still discussing exercising, consider getting yourself a personal trainer. That way, you can get the most out of your exercises, and your trainer also doubles as an exercise partner as well because they hold you accountable for your commitments. Your trainer is very helpful when you do strength training because they can teach you how to perform the exercise with the correct form and to prevent you from injuring yourself.

Rely Less on Convenience Foods

Convenient foods are convenient but not healthy. Not by a long shot. They are rich in calories and often do not pack essential nutrients such as protein, fiber, vitamins, etc. If you can, ditch inconvenient foods altogether.

Find an Activity you Enjoy

When you have done enough exercise, you will know what activities you like. One way to encourage yourself to exercise more regularly is by making it entertaining than a chore. If possible, stick to your favorite activities, and you can get the most out of your exercises. Keep in mind that the activities you enjoy may not be effective or needed, so you need to find other exercises to compensate, which you may not enjoy so much. For instance, if you like jogging, then you can work your leg muscles, but your arms are not involved. So you need to do pushups or other strength training exercises.

Here, your trainer can help you decide and create a workout routine that you can stick with as well.

CHAPTER 13 - TIPS ON LOSING WEIGHT ON KETO AFTER 50

Check with a Healthcare Provider

As mentioned earlier, the keto diet works for many people, but it isn't for everyone. Your dietitian can tell you whether keto diet would work. However, it helps to check in with your healthcare provider to ensure that you do not have any medical condition that prevents you from losing weight, such as hypothyroidism and polycystic ovarian syndrome. It helps to know well in advance whether your body is even capable of losing fat in the first place before you commit and see no result, right?

Eat Less at Night

While the science still argues about it to this day, it seems more logical that breakfast is the most important meal of the day considering that you would not have eaten for the past 8 hours whereas the interval between breakfast and lunch, and lunch and dinner is 5 or 6 hours at best. Dinner should be small because your body does not need to expend that much energy when you are sleeping anyway. So the excess energy becomes fat.

So keep dinner light. For one, it helps you lose weight. Another reason is if you have a heavy dinner, your body will strain itself trying to digest everything. That means your body would remain active until all the food is digested, meaning that you will not get restful sleep if you can sleep at all.

Bottom line: Eat light and eat dinner at least 4 hours before bedtime. Any sooner and you will have a hard time sleeping.

BODY COMPOSITION

Your body isn't just "weight" alone. Your body is composed of fat, muscles, fluid, bones, etc. What you want to lose is fat weight, not muscle weight or fluid weight. You want as little fat mass in your body as possible while still maintaining a healthy level of non-fat mass in your body. There are many ways you can measure your body fat, but the simplest method is to measure your calves, thighs, waist, chest, and biceps.

HYDRATE PROPERLY

That means drinking enough water or herbal tea and ditch sweetened beverages or other drinks that contain sugar altogether. Making the transition will be difficult for the first few weeks, but your body will be thanking you for it. There is nothing healthier than good old plain water, and the recommended amount is 2 gallons a day. However, because you are on a keto diet, your body needs to use up more water, so consider 2 gallons to the absolute minimum amount of water you need to drinks. I recommend you drink between 3 or even 4 gallons a day when you are on a keto diet. If you get thirsty, then it is a sign of dehydration, so drink some water. Drinking plenty of water also leads to additional calories burned. You can shave off a few more calories by drinking cold water because your body will spend more energy trying to regulate your body temperature.

SUPPLEMENTS

When you get older, your body starts to lose its ability to absorb certain nutrients, which leads to deficits. For example, vitamin B12 and

CHAPTER 13 - TIPS ON LOSING WEIGHT ON KETO AFTER 50

folate are some of the most common nutrients that people over 50 lack. They have an impact on your mood, energy level, and weight loss rate.

Therefore, if you feel tired when you are on your keto diet, perhaps you do not get enough nutrients that your body needs. That does not mean you should eat more, no. You just need to take the right supplements.

Get Enough Sleep

When you are over 50, your body starts to fail you. You no longer have the ability to party past midnight without feeling horrible for the rest of the month. If there is the most crucial time to get 8 hours of sleep a day, then it is right now.

Getting enough sleep helps your body regulate the hormones in your body, so try to aim for 7 to 9 hours of sleep a day. You can get more restful sleep by creating a nighttime routine that involves not looking at a computer, phone, or TV screen for at least 1 hour before bed. You can drink warm milk or water to help your body relax or even do 10 to 20 minutes of stretching so you can get a restful sleep.

While we are on the subject of sleeping, try to maintain a consistent sleeping schedule. I understand that you want to sleep and wake up 1 to 4 hours later than usual during the weekend. But you want to go to bed and wake up at the same time, your mood and energy level will be higher. An added benefit is that your body will learn to wake up on its own even without the alarm.

Mindful Eating

Mindfulness isn't restricted to meditation alone. Again, we will not go over meditation in this guidebook because it is another topic altogether. But what you can do here is learn to love and appreciate your food. It sounds obnoxious, but it helps your mood and promotes weight loss.

Simply put, you just have to put away your phone and take away any other sources of distractions and focus solely on your food, how it tastes, etc. That means eating slowly. You will learn to appreciate how tasty your food is because you focus on eating.

How does this translate to weight loss? You see, there is a system in your body that determines how full you are. The issue here is that this system is not instantaneous. It takes some time to measure how full your stomach it before sending the signal to your brain. So when you eat too quickly, by the time you feel full, you would have already overshot by a country mile. If you eat slowly, your body has enough time to register your fullness bite by bite. So when you feel full, you have not overeaten.

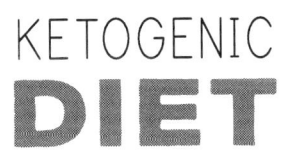

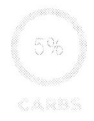

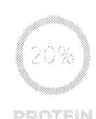

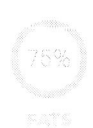

CHAPTER 14

CONCLUSION

Chapter 14 - Conclusion

Now that you are familiar with the Keto diet on many levels, you should feel confident in your ability to start your own Keto journey. This diet plan isn't going to hinder you or limit you, so do your best to keep this in mind as you begin changing your lifestyle and adjusting your eating habits. Packed with good fats and plenty of protein, your body is going to go through a transformation as it works to see these things as energy. Before you know it, your body will have an automatically accessible reserve that you can utilize at any time. Whether you need a boost of energy first thing in the morning or a second wind to keep you going throughout the day, this will already be inside of you.

As you take care of yourself through the next few years, you can feel great knowing that the Keto diet aligns with the anti-aging lifestyle that you seek. Not only does it keep you looking great and feeling younger, but it also acts as a preventative barrier from various ailments and conditions. The body tends to weaken as you age, but Keto helps to keep a shield up in front of it by giving you plenty of opportunities to burn energy and create muscle mass. Instead of taking the things that you need to feel great, Keto only takes what you have in abundance. This is how you will always end up feeling your best each day.

Arguably one of the best diets around, Keto keeps you feeling so great because you have many meal options! There is no shortage of delicious and filling meals that you can eat while you are on any of the Keto diet plans. You can even take this diet with you as you eat out at restaurants and friends' houses. As long as you can remember the simple guidelines, you should have no problems staying on track with Keto. Cravings become almost non-existent as your body works to change the way it digests. Instead of relying on glucose in your bloodstream, your body switches focus. It begins using fat as soon as you reach the state of ketosis that you are aiming for. The best part is, you do not have to do anything other than eating within your fat/protein/carb percentages. Your body will do the rest on its own.

Because this is a way that your body can properly function for long periods, Keto is proven to be more than a simple fad diet. Originating with a medical background for helping epilepsy patients, the Keto diet has been tried and tested for decades. Many successful studies align with the knowledge that Keto works. Whether you are trying to be on a diet for a month or a year, both are just as healthy for you. Keto is an adjustment, but it is one that will continue benefiting you for as long as you are able to keep it up. Good luck on your journey ahead!